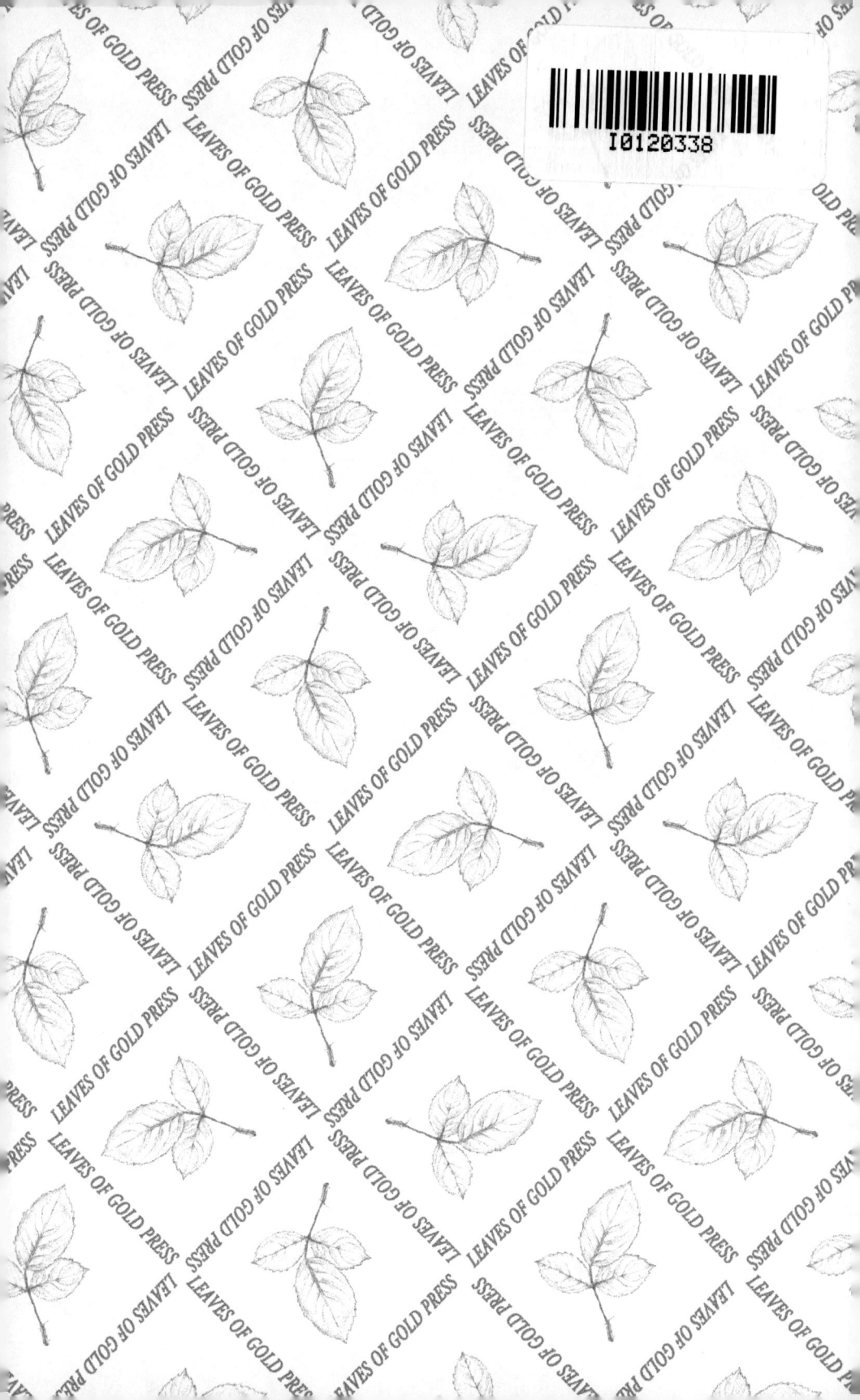

Ultimate Beauty 2024

#2 Hair, Body & Smile

Creator: Reed, Elizabeth M., author.

Title: Ultimate beauty 2024 : #2 hair, body and smile / Elizabeth M. Reed.
ISBN: 9781923212114 (paperback)
Series: Ultimate beauty ; 2.
Notes: Includes index.

Subjects: Teeth--Care and hygiene.
Hair--Care and hygiene.
Cosmetics.
Beauty, Personal.
Surgery, Plastic.

Dewey Number: 646.7

Leaves of Gold Press

ABN 67 099 575 078
PO Box 345, Shoreham, 3916, Victoria, Australia
www.leavesofgoldpress.com

Ultimate Beauty 2024

#2 Hair, Body & Smile

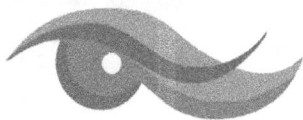

Elizabeth M. Reed, B.A. (Hons) Dip. Ed.

Other books in this series:

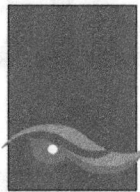

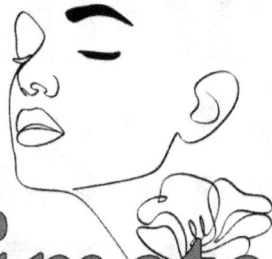

Ultimate Beauty

#1 2024

Face and Skin

Elizabeth M. Reed, B.A. (Hons) Dip. Ed.

Contents

Legend

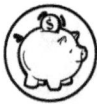

Frugal: Economical ways of achieving cosmetic improvements.

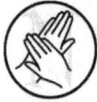

Non-surgical: Cosmetic techniques in which no instruments penetrate the skin.

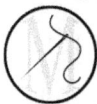

Minimally-invasive: Cosmetic techniques that involve minor incisions with surgical instruments but usually require no general anesthesia.

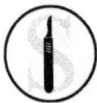

Surgical: Cosmetic techniques that involve an incision with surgical instruments.

FOREWORD

Most of us want to look our best, just like all those 'ageless' movie stars. Finding the perfect cosmetic treatment, however, can be confusing. What treatments are available? Which of them best suits your needs and budget?

Hunting down all your options, finding conveniently located salons or clinics and reading reviews from other clients all takes time.

For your convenience, the 'Ultimate Beauty' series of books helps to solve the problem. We make the job of finding the appropriate cosmetic treatments quick and easy, for both men and women. Dozens of beauty techniques have been described and compared for you, so that you can find the most suitable therapy available.

THE EASY GUIDE TO CHOOSING

It is sometimes difficult to find information about ways to improve your appearance. Every day, thousands of people are having cosmetic enhancements, but most of them prefer to keep that fact secret, and avoid talking about it.

In this series '*Ultimate Beauty: Books 1 and 2*', we compare the latest cosmetic treatments, techniques and procedures.

The aim is to provide you with the convenience of comparison and the benefit of explanatory articles.

Armed with this information, you will be in the best position to evaluate your cosmetic treatment requirements.

This enables you to avoid spending your time calling or visiting numerous salons and clinics to compare treatments and products with often-confusing brand names. It also helps you find a treatment or product better suited to your needs, at a given price point.

RETURN TO THE 'YOU' YOU KNEW

People have been enhancing their looks with potions, lotions, plucking, shaving, dyes, powders, paints, tattoos, corsets, wigs, jewelry and so on since the dawn of the human race. In the 21st century, more sophisticated cosmetic treatments are undergoing a surge of popularity throughout the world.

There are many reasons why people seek cosmetic treatments. Skin blemishes such as acne, eczema, spider veins and rosacea can cause people to feel uncomfortable in social situations. Excess hair on the face or body can be embarrassing, too. As we age, our skin loses elasticity and may sustain sun damage, leading to wrinkles, pigmentation and sagging. Dieting alone may not remove fat deposits from certain areas of the body, such as the hips, belly or upper arms. This is where techniques such as liposuction or non-invasive fat treatments may be useful.

We all want to look our best, and these days there are many safe, quick rejuvenating and skin tightening therapies available.

Numerous appearance-enhancement techniques are now being offered. The range of choices might surprise you – for instance, many people might think that loss of eyebrow hair cannot be redressed; however there is even a way of making eyebrows appear thick again, and shaping them to flatter your face. Another procedure, cosmetic tattooing, is a way of applying semi-permanent makeup, so that you don't have to apply eyeliner or mascara every day. There are even non-surgical treatments for patchy baldness.

More and more non-surgical cosmetic techniques are now being offered. It is no longer necessary to 'go under the knife' to achieve improvements.

COMPARE COSMETIC TREATMENTS.

When – or if – you decide you are ready to rejuvenate your appearance with something more than over-the-counter or home-made cosmetic treatments, where do you start to look? There is an enormous and bewildering array of possibilities offered by an ever-burgeoning number of clinics and salons. Which technique is best for your particular needs?

That is the question these books strive to answer. They provide you with the information needed to compare cosmetic treatments so that you can make an educated choice.

In describing these treatments, all efforts have been made to be objective and unbiased. A broad description of each technique is given, without elaboration on details.

These books do not recommend any particular cosmetic treatments and it is up to the consumer to consult their practitioner on associated topics such as psychological issues, side-effects, contraindications, possible discomfort, cost and after-treatment care.

Welcome to these pages. Enjoy browsing!

Elizabeth M. Reed

(P.S. This volume contains a bonus section on nails!)

Search for cruelty-free cosmetics online. Scan this QR code with any scanning app on your phone or other device.

Cruelty-Free
Beauty Products

We recommend that you always choose to buy cruelty-free beauty products. They can be identified by this symbol.

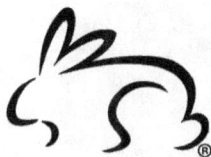

Testing products on animals is not merely a matter of dabbing some nail polish on a rabbit's claws, or wiping some shampoo on a beagle's ears. I will not distress readers by describing exactly how beauty products are tested on animals. Suffice to say that animal testing laboratories are torture chambers where horrific practices are carried out. If you wish, you can find out more here.

www.peta.org/issues/
animals-used-for-experimentation/
Seek cruelty-free cosmetics here:
https://crueltyfree.peta.org/

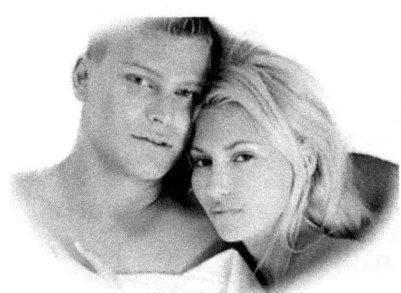

INTRODUCTION

WHY DO WE WANT TO LOOK GOOD?

As I wrote in the introduction to the companion book *'Ultimate Beauty 1: Face and Skin'*, most men and women would say that when they look good, they feel good. Scientists tell us that human beings are 'hard-wired' to be attracted to good-looking people. Feeling attractive to others can boost our self-esteem.

Human beings are social animals and by our very nature, it is essential to us to feel accepted and loved; even admired. All in all, life generally seems better when you look your best.

Physically attractive men and women are more successful in dating, landing a job and being elected.[1] [2] [3] In social
situations, other people are more likely to support them.[4]
They receive lighter sentences in courts and are viewed
as being friendlier. Unfortunately, beauty can indeed be
discriminatory.

Looking good may make you appear not only more
desirable, but also cleverer and more virtuous. In many cases,
humans attribute positive characteristics, such as intelligence and honesty, to physically attractive people without
consciously realizing it.[5] From research done in the United
States and United Kingdom, it was found that men (more
than women), tend to think that people who are physically
attractive are also more intelligent.[6]

---

1   Berscheid E, Dion K (1971) Physical attractiveness and dating choice: A
test of the matching hypothesis. J Exp Soc Psychol 7: 173–189. doi: 10.1016/0022-
1031(71)90065-5
2   Cross JF, Cross J (1971) Age, sex, race, and the perception of facial beauty.
Dev Psychol 5: 433–439. doi: 10.1037/h0031591
3   Barber N (1995) The evolutionary psychology of physical attractiveness:
Sexual selection and human morphology. Ethology and Sociobiology 16: 395–424.
doi: 10.1016/0162-3095(95)00068-2
4   Sarason BR, Sarason IG, Hacker TA, Basham RB (1985) Concomitants
of social support: Social skills, physical attractiveness, and gender. J Pers Soc Psychol
49: 469–480. doi: 10.1037/0022-3514.49.2.469
5   Dion K, Berscheid E, Walster E (December 1972). "What is beautiful is good". J Pers Soc Psychol 24 (3): 285–90. doi:10.1037/h0033731. PMID
4655540.
6   Kanazawa Satoshi (2011). "Intelligence and physical attractiveness". Intelligence 39 (1): 7–14. doi:10.1016/j. intell. 2010.11.003

WHAT IS BEAUTY?

Scientists view beauty as an evolutionary sexual strategy. Beauty usually indicates good health. It is like an advertisement declaring, 'I am healthy; therefore I am a good candidate to pass on your genes.'

Attractiveness is closely associated with physical characteristics such as facial features, body shape, voice and hair.[7]

Research shows that even human babies can judge appearance as attractive or unattractive.

Some beauty fashions come and go – hairstyles are a good example of that – but our basic idea of beauty, which crosses the boundaries of culture and race, is not arbitrary. Beauty has a function, and that function is hard-wired into the brain. Beauty, defined as 'fitness to mate', is also of vital importance to most other animals – not just humans.

Men generally prefer women with smooth, evenly-colored skin, large eyes, curvaceous bodies, and full lips. All these characteristics are clues to youth, vibrant health, and fertility. Lips, for example, become plumper when there is plenty of estrogen in the body; they are fullest when girls reach puberty and begin to be fertile. When women reach menopause and lose fertility, their lips lose their volume, as well as some of their color. Unblemished, even skin tone signals youth, because as we age our skin often exhibits the discolorations of sun damage. It is also an indicator of good health, because skin lesions can be a symptom of underlying disease.

7   Barber N (1995) The evolutionary psychology of physical attractiveness: Sexual selection and human morphology. Ethology and Sociobiology 16: 395–424. doi: 10.1016/0162-3095(95)00068-2

Is it bad to want to look good?

If the quest for beauty becomes an obsession, then it can be destructive; however, paying attention to the way we look can be good for us. Attention to personal grooming is one indicator that a person is in a positive frame of mind. When people become depressed, they usually lose interest in their appearance.

An interest in beauty and its fashions is not as 'shallow' as some people claim. We benefit psychologically from transforming ourselves, in dressing up and putting on makeup for special occasions, just as tribal societies have, for millennia, adorned themselves with body paint and feathers for similar reasons.

WHAT MAKES A BODY ATTRACTIVE?

There has been plenty of research into this subject. A number of factors come into play when we try to divine the sources of physical attractiveness. Some of them include:

- Symmetry
- Smooth skin and even skin color
- The degree of sexual dimorphism (the differences in appearance between men and women)
- The appearance of the hair and teeth
- Certain proportions

Symmetry
Scientists have found that when people are looking for a mate, their assessment of physical beauty depends largely upon symmetry. The more symmetrical a person's body is,

the more attractive that person is to members of the opposite sex.[8]

Human beings are drawn to symmetry in nature. For example if asked to choose between eating an apple that is lop-sided and an apple that is symmetrical, the overwhelming majority of people will choose the symmetrical apple. We sense a 'wrongness' about the misshapen fruit.

'In animals [or plants] with two sides that were designed by natural selection to be symmetrical, subtle departures from symmetry may reflect poor development or exposure to environmental or genetic stress. In many species these departures are related to poor health, lower survival, and fewer offspring.' [9]

Both facial symmetry and body symmetry are considered more beautiful by observers. Symmetrical proportions are deemed to be signs of biological fitness.

Women view physically symmetrical men as more attractive, and men whose body and face shape is symmetrical tend to have more female sexual partners.[10] This holds true regardless of race or culture.

Any differences in left-right symmetry are often so subtle as to be virtually undetectable; a slightly wider nostril on one side, for example; or a tiny chip missing from one front tooth. In most cases, the differences between the left and right sides of a person's body are miniscule—only about one

8   *Symmetrical Bodies Are More Beautiful to Humans. Ker Than, for National Geographic News. August 18, 2008*

9   *Brown, W.M. (2012). Symmetry and evolution: A genomic antagonism approach. In Filomena de Sousa and Gonzalo Munévar (Editors) Sex, Reproduction and Darwinism. Pickering & Chatto Publishers: London.*

10   *The relationship between shape symmetry and perceived skin condition in male facial attractiveness. B.C. Jones, A.C. Little, D.R. Feinberg, I.S. Penton-Voak, B.P. Tiddeman, D.I. Perrett. Evolution and Human Behavior 25 (2004) 24–30*

to three percent.[11] Yet we are hard-wired to notice them, almost unconsciously, and to find symmetrical bodies more attractive.

There also appears to be a strong correlation between body symmetry and body characteristics that are sex-typical. Remarkably, scientists report that men who possess physical characteristics usually viewed as 'masculine'—for example greater height, broader shoulders, and smaller hip-to-waist ratios— were also more likely to have more symmetrical bodies.

Likewise, women whose bodies were more symmetrical were inclined to exhibit a greater number of 'feminine' traits, such as longer and more slender legs, and larger breasts.

According to J. T. Manning of the University of Liverpool, U.K., 'This means a woman who pairs with a man with a masculine body or a man who chooses a woman with a feminine body is likely to get a symmetric partner with all the associated fitness benefits.'

Smooth skin and even skin color

As I wrote in 'Ultimate Beauty 1: Face and Skin' – 'It's not just symmetry and averageness that make faces attractive. A luminous, unblemished complexion is another factor. Smooth, evenly-colored skin in both sexes gives the impression of youth and good health.

'Conversely blotches, discolored patches, blemishes and lesions signal poor health or aging. This is why foundation and cover-up makeup play a big part in making women look more attractive.

---

11   Manning, JT, RL Trivers, D Singh, R Thornhill. The mystery of female beauty. Nature. 1999 (399): 214-215.

'"Both skin topography (smoothness or bumpiness) and skin coloration affect the perception of facial age, health and attractiveness," says researcher B. Fink. "Skin topography seems to be a strong age cue while skin coloration is a stronger predictor of facial health perception."[12]

'When we're young and healthy, our skin is flawless. But as we get older, our skin tends to discolor and lose its smooth texture, whether from sun damage, scars or other kinds of injury. It is no surprise that concealing such imperfections makes us look younger and healthier.

'Consciously or not, we all use skin appearance to make judgments about a person's health. In the study cited, researchers cropped photographs of cheek skin from 170 women and girls, aged 11 to 76. They asked 353 men and women to rate each cheek sample for attractiveness, health and youth. They also asked them to guess (based on nothing more than a cheek image) the age of the person in the photograph.[13]

'Raters' guesses about the ages of the subjects tended to be accurate. The older the subject of the photograph, the less likely they were to be rated healthy, attractive and youthful. Nonetheless, one factor defeated age: The skin samples with even tone and texture were rated as younger, healthier and more attractive. Smooth, even skin tone and texture are signs of good health and minimal sun damage. No wonder human beings find it attractive.

---

12   Fink B1, Matts PJ. J Eur Acad Dermatol Venereol. 2008 Apr;22(4):493-8. Epub 2007 Dec 13. The effects of skin color distribution and topography cues on the perception of female facial age and health.
13   Color homogeneity and visual perception of age, health, and attractiveness of female facial skin. P. J. Matts, B. Fink, K. Grammer and M. Burquest. Journal of the American Academy of Dermatology, Vol. 57, pp.977-984, 2007

'For the survival of the species human beings are 'wired' to see skin free from acne, pigmentation disorders or other dermatological issues as indicating healthy genes, and hence better chances of begetting healthy offspring.

'The good news is, you have some control over this issue. Your diet and lifestyle play a more vital role in your skin's appearance than even your genetic inheritance. If you want to have even skin tone, wear sunscreen. Most uneven skin color is caused by sun damage. Daily application of sunblock (preferably a zinc oxide formula) is your best protection. For an extra boost to your skin tone, choose foods containing carotenoids, such as carrots, sweet potatoes, spinach, kale, collard greens and tomatoes.'

ATTRACTIVENESS VS BEAUTY

Beauty does not automatically mean attractiveness. We are attracted to people for a wide range of reasons that go beyond their skin texture or bone structure. Attractiveness is more than just finding someone physically appealing.

If it's evolution that drives us, why can't we all simply agree on who is beautiful and who is not? When you talk about individuals, it gets a little more complicated. Evolution explains why we find certain attributes attractive—to a degree. Factors like voice, facial expression, body language, personality and even scent also enhance one's appeal, meaning physical features only take you so far before your inner beauty shines through.

Physical attraction may play a significant role when we first meet someone, but there is more to attraction than meets the eye. Simply being friendly and nice plays an important part in attraction. People who aren't stereotypically good-looking appear attractive to those who know and like them. Researchers asked subjects to evaluate each other before and after working together in groups. In general, likeable people were described as more beautiful because of their happy persona.

Beyond kindness, other traits that make people attractive are cooperativeness and a sense of humor. Being friendly and out-going and making an effort to get along with others all go a long way towards making you seem more attractive to others whilst also boosting the quality of your relationships.

People who can communicate in an expressive and animated way tend to be more liked compared with those who are difficult-to-read. This is because we are more confident in our reading of them and they are therefore less of a threat.

Research shows that two people who share similar interests, values, likes and dislikes feel drawn to each other. People can also feel attracted to others who share a similar physical appearance, background, or personality.

Psychology professor Albert Mehrabian suggested that there are three important elements that account differently for our liking of a person. He calls these as the 'three Vs' – verbal, vocal and visual.[14]

Mehrabian postulated that 93% of expression is non-verbal. Our actual words make up only 7% of communication, while 38% comes from tone of voice, and 55% comes from our body language. One more element, however, does play a part in our attractiveness to other human beings, and that is smell.

---

14   Swami, V., and Furnham, A. (2008). *The Psychology of physical attraction*. London: Routledge.

Smell and attractiveness

Certain body odors are connected to human sexual attraction, according to research. Again, this relates back to the innate drive to perpetuate the human race. Subconsciously, by way of scent, humans can discern whether a potential mate will pass on favorable genetic traits to their offspring.

'Research on human mating has found that the effect of scent on males and on females differs[15]. Part of this difference is caused by the different motives each gender holds for mating. Males, in order to pass on genes, subconsciously notice and are attracted to traits that indicate fertility in females, such as a voice of higher pitch, a specific hip-to-waist ratio, and a certain body odor. Evolutionarily, females have two main motives for mating: to pass on genes and to find a partner who can provide adequate support for herself and future offspring. As a female reaches the fertile stage of her menstrual cycle, the desire to pass on favorable traits to offspring gains more importance and the female becomes more attracted than usual to males with favorable traits. Many such traits are subliminally detected through scent.'[16]

Evolutionary biologist Randy Thornhill of the University of New Mexico found that men with symmetrical facial features even smell better to women. In some cases, women in Thornhill's study reported that they could not smell anything on a man's sweaty shirt, yet they were, nonetheless,

---

15   *Haselton, Martie G.; Gangestad, Steven W. (2006). "Conditional expression of women's desires and men's mate guarding across the ovulatory cycle". Hormones and Behavior 49 (4): 509–518. doi:10.1016/j.yhbeh.2005.10.006. PMID 16403409.*

16   *'Body odor and subconscious human sexual attraction.' Wikipedia. Retrieved 28th October 2014*

attracted to it. 'We think the detection of these types of scent is way outside consciousness', Thornhill said.

This attraction to scent goes beyond pheremones. Scientific American journalist Adam Hadhazy writes, 'Humans might use a nuanced concoction of chemicals even more complex than formal pheromones to attract potential mates.' [17]

If this is so, then men who wish to be attractive to women might do better to refrain from using 'masculine fragrances' such as after-shave!

Kate Fox writes: 'Widely publicized research findings on female sensitivity to male pheromones have also led some men to believe that the odor of their natural sweat is highly attractive to women.

'Women are indeed highly sensitive to male pheromones, particularly around ovulation, but many popular assumptions about the effects of these pheromones are the result of misinterpretation and over-simplification of the research results.

'All male pheromones are not equally attractive, and some of the myths stem from an understandable confusion over their names. The male pheromone *androstenone* is not the same as *androstenol*. Androstenol is the scent produced by fresh male sweat, and is attractive to females. Androstenone is produced by male sweat after exposure to oxygen – i.e. when less fresh – and is perceived as highly unpleasant by females (except during ovulation, when their responses change from 'negative' to 'neutral').

'So, men who believe that their 'macho', sweaty body-odor is attractive to women are deluding themselves,

17   *'Do Pheromones Play a Role in Our Sex Lives?' By Adam Hadhazy. Scientific American. February 13, 2012.*

unless they are constantly producing fresh sweat and either naked or changing their clothes every 20 minutes to remove any trace of the oxidized sweat.'[18]

Everyone has a different opinion as to what smells are pleasing. Some tribes prefer the smell of cows, or the small of onions, to any other.[19] The sense of smell is powerful and primitive. Smells can evoke and vivid images and emotions and even influence people's moods. Unconsciously, we can even be attracted to the smell of people with the same political beliefs![20]

The section of the human brain that interprets smell is in the brain's limbic system, an area so intimately entwined with memory and feeling that it is sometimes referred to as the 'emotional brain'. In spite of this biological wiring, however, smells would not awaken memories and emotions if we did accumulate learned responses. The first time you smell a new scent, you (consciously or unconsciously) associate it with an experience, a person, an object or even an instant in time. Your brain creates a link between the smell and a memory; for example associating the smell of lavender with your grandmother, or a certain aftershave with a school principal you disliked, or the smell of sunscreen with the beach. When you experience the smell again, the connection awakens that particular memory or mood. Lavender might call up a specific grandmother-related memory or simply

18   Fox, Kate. "The Smell Report." Social Issues Research Centre. (Sept. 20, 2010). http://www.sirc.org/publik/smell.pdf
19   ibid.
20   Assortative Mating on Ideology Could Operate Through Olfactory Cues. Rose McDermott, Dustin Tingley and Peter K. Hatemi. American Journal of Political Science, Volume 58, Issue 4, pages 997–1005, October 2014. DOI: 10.1111/ajps.12133 ©2014, Midwest Political Science Association

make you feel content. A whiff of aftershave might make you feel anxious or angry without your understanding the reason. This partly explains why people have different preferences in smells. One of my friends finds herself attracted to men who smell of machine oil, because during her teens she happily dated a youth whose hobby was tinkering with his motor-bike!

Because it is during our youth that we experience most new smells, odors frequently awaken childhood memories. The fact is, however, that we actually start to link smells and emotion even before we are born! Infants who were exposed to certain smells when they were still embryos in the womb, show a liking for the smells.[21]

It is difficult to know what memories, emotions or cultural responses certain external smells can call up in other people. One thing is for certain however: our own personal—clean and hygienic—natural odor, whether or not we are conscious of its existence, is going to be attractive to numerous people, and not infrequently. So avoid the strong perfumes—you may be masking your own subtle, attractive, natural scent!

In conclusion: we can change our appearance with makeup and cosmetic procedures, with manipulation of our body and scalp hair; with clothing, tattoos and adornments; but appearance is only part of the story. Of all the elements that make us attractive to others, beauty is only one.

---

21   'Long-term flavor recognition in humans with prenatal garlic experience'. Peter G. Hepper1, Deborah L. Wells, James C. Dornan and Catherine Lynch. DOI: 10.1002/dev.21059 Copyright © 2012 Wiley Periodicals, Inc. Developmental Psychobiology, Volume 55, Issue 5, pages 568–574, July 2013

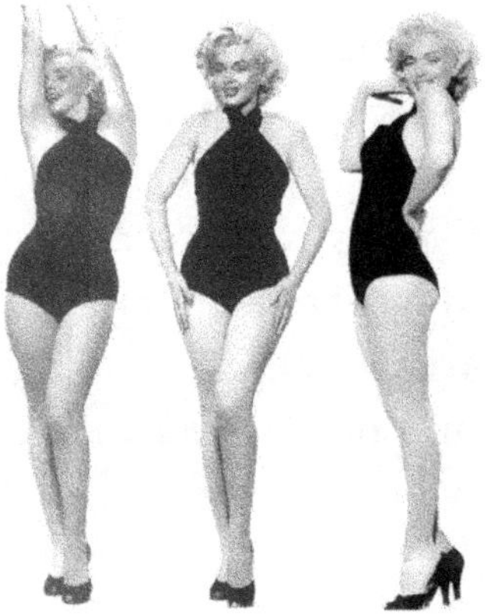

Part 1:
Body Issues

BODY ISSUES

WOMEN'S BODY SHAPE

Most human cultures value female beauty more than male physical attractiveness.[22] In terms of evolutionary psychology, this is probably because women's bodies are more intimately and extensively involved with child-bearing and child-rearing.

Some studies have shown that heterosexual men from different cultures all over the world are – consciously or unconsciously – more attracted to women with a waist-to-hip ratio of 0.7; that is, when the waist's width is about 70% of the hips' width.[23]

Once again, this relates to beauty's evolutionary sexual strategy. Evolutionary psychologists explain that the 0.7 waist-to-hip ratio indicates that a woman is better suited for bearing children.[24] In other words, her hips are the optimum size for giving birth to healthy babies.

---

22   Margaret F. Braun, Portland State University. Angela Bryan, University of Colorado at Boulder. Female waist-to-hip and male waist-to-shoulder ratios as determinants of romantic partner desirability. . Journal of Social and Personal Relationships.

23   Singh, D., Dixson, B. J., Jessop, T. S., Morgan, B. B., & Dixson, A. F. (2010). Cross-cultural consensus for waist–hip ratio and women's attractiveness. Evolution and Human Behavior, 31 (3), 176–81. doi:10.1016/j.evolhumbehav.2009.09.001

24   Singh, D., & Singh, D. (2011). Shape and significance of feminine beauty: An evolutionary perspective. Sex Roles, 64(9-10), 723-731. doi:10.1007/s11199-011-9938-z

'Waist-to-hip-ratio (WHR) is a phenotypic cue to fertility, fecundity, neurodevelopmental resources in offspring, and overall health, and is indicative of "good genes" in women.'[25]

'Hourglass' figures announce 'reproductive capability,' which is why, whether or not they are aware of it, hetero-sexual, virile males find these attributes attractive in females.

A woman's waist-to-hip ratio, and its subsequent effect on her attractiveness in the eyes of men, may affect her sexual behavior. Women close to the magical 0.7 have been shown to have more sexual partners, to begin sexual relationships at an earlier age, and to be more likely to cheat on their partner.[26]

Women with a waist-to-hip ratio close to 0.7 have curvaceous figures. As the ratio climbs toward 0.8 and 0.9 (i.e. either the hips become narrower or the waist becomes wider), the overall body shape tends to become more cylindri-cal and less curvy. Men, for example, who are typically far from curvaceous, usually have waist-to-hip ratios close to 0.9.

Researchers claim that the significance of the waist-to-hip ratio is that it holds true for bodies of different sizes. Across the globe the average overall female body size can vary a great deal; nonetheless, they say, men find the same ratio attractive.

---

25   Steven M. Platek, Devendra Singh. Optimal Waist-to-Hip Ratios in Women Activate Neural Reward Centers in Men. Published: February 05, 2010. DOI: 10.1371/journal.pone.0009042

26   Singh, D. (1993). Adaptive significance of female physical attractiveness: Role of waist-to-hip ratio. Journal of Personality and Social Psychology, 65(2), 293–307. doi:10.1037/0022-3514.65.2.293

Some declare that this holds true for the past as well as the present. Researchers analyzed the waist-to-hip ratio of Playboy centerfolds and Miss America winners, dating back to the 1920s.[27] They found that men's preference for the 0.7 ratio remained the same, regardless of the prevailing fashion in body size. The belles they studied ranged from Marilyn Monroe, who by today's standards would be considered 'large', to Twiggy, the ultra-thin teenage model who became an international fashion icon during the 1960s.

Despite the body size of these belles decreasing over the decades, the waist-to-hip ratio remained about the same. Slender or voluptuous, they all had similar waist-to-hip proportions.

The researchers deduced that women's attractiveness to men is not concerned so much with body weight as it is about how that weight is distributed. This implies that women do not have to starve themselves or exercise incessantly to be attractive to the opposite sex.

Scientist Devendra Singh's studies show that when men rate the attractiveness of silhouettes of women's bodies, they usually pick the silhouette associated with the healthiest weight for women — neither too slender, nor too fat.[28]

The 'ideal' body shape can be a cultural construct.

27   Singh, D. (1993). Adaptive significance of female physical attractiveness: Role of waist-to-hip ratio. Journal of Personality and Social Psychology, 65(2), 293–307. doi:10.1037/0022-3514.65.2.293

28   Psychological Topics 15 (2006), 2, 331-350 Original Scientific Article – UDC 159.9.015.7.072 572.51-055.2. Role of Body Fat and Body Shape on Judgment of Female Health and Attractiveness: An Evolutionary Perspective Devendra Singh, University of Texas at Austin, Department of Psychology. Dorian Singh, Oxford University Department of Social Policy and Social Work.

BODY ISSUES

The instinct to choose fit and fertile partners has been fine-tuned over a hundred thousand years of evolutionary selection; however biology does not explain everything. The desire to procreate is not the only drive that influences our standards of beauty.

Douglas Yu, a biologist from Great Britain, and Glenn Shepard, an anthropologist at the University of California at Berkeley, found that among some indigenous peoples of Peru, males preferred women with a higher waist-to-hip ratio than that which is preferred in Western cultures.[29]

There is some scientific debate about whether the 0.7 ratio 'hourglass' figure is a universal truth which applies cross-culturally.[30] The hormones that make women physically stronger and better able to manage stress are also likely to reposition body-fat from the hips to the waist. Therefore, in cases like the Peruvian situation, where women have to be good providers and protectors, they may be less likely to have the 0.7 ratio 'hourglass' figure.

MEN'S BODY SHAPE

As discussed, science has shown that in general, hetero-sexual human beings tend to perceive beauty in members of the opposite sex who exhibit reproductive potential.

For females, the signs of a potentially good male mate include:

- Facial symmetry
- Body symmetry
- Greater height

29   Nature 396, 321-322 (26 November 1998) | doi:10.1038/24512. Is beauty in the eye of the beholder? Douglas W. Yu & Glenn H. Shepard, Jr
30   Waist-to-Hip Ratio across Cultures: Trade-Offs between Androgen- and Estrogen-Dependent Traits. Elizabeh Cashdan, Department of Anthropology, University of Utah. Chicago Journals, Current Anthropology Vol. 49, No. 6, December 2008.

- Broader shoulders
- Smaller differences between the measurements of waist and hips
- Larger differences between the measurements of shoulders and waist.[31]
- Facial masculinity (A 'masculine face' has a relatively pronounced chin, strong jaw, narrow eyes and well-defined brow.[32])

Waist-to-hip ratio: Studies show that women rate waist-to-hip ratios for men between 0.85 and 0.95 as most attractive, with 0.9 being the most attractive. This indicates a body shape in which there is only a small difference between the waist size and the hip size.

Shoulder-to-waist ratio: Women also prefer the looks of men with broad shoulders and a relatively small waist. A low shoulder-to-waist ratio signifies a tapering 'V' body shape with broader shoulders and a narrower waist. A man with these body characteristics might be viewed as physically stronger, and thus more able to protect a partner and children.[33]

'In addition to preferring tall, symmetrical men... women may prefer a body shape that conveys information about

---

31   *Optimal Waist-to-Hip Ratios in Women Activate Neural Reward Centers in Men. Steven M. Platek mail, Devendra Singh. Published: February 05, 2010* DOI: 10.1371/journal.pone.0009042

32   *Fertile women want macho-looking men: Effect is more pronounced among women partnered with less-masculine-looking men, researchers find; male intelligence shows no such effect. By Clint Talbott. Colorado Arts & Sciences Magazine. Date unknown.*

33   *Franzoi, S. L., & Herzog, M. E. (1987). Judging physical attractiveness: What body aspects do we use? Personality and Social Psychology Bulletin, 13 (1), 19–33.*

a man's dominance in the form of strength and ability to protect. We suspect that a body shape with broad shoulders and a narrow waist and hips will be optimally desirable to women.'[34]

Height: Researchers have computed the ratio of height difference that heterosexual women (usually subliminally) seek in a potential partner. When they were presented with pictures of men and women standing next to each other, women tended to be drawn to men who were 1.09 times taller than the female.

Physical fitness: 'The strength of the attractiveness-fitness relationship ... suggests that signaling physical fitness may be one of the key functions of male attractiveness.' [35]

Scent: Researchers have discovered that women rated a man's scent as more attractive the more his major histocompatibility complex (MHC) differed from hers. Scientists surmise that nature has created this association because the children of people with very different MHC sets may be blessed with stronger immune systems.

Sound: Women preferred men with deeper voices. One study found that 'Deep male voices ... were judged [by women] as more attractive because they conveyed that the speaker had a large frame—but were found to be most

34   Hughes, S. M., & Gallup, G. G. (2003). Sex differences in morphological predictors of sexual behavior: Shoulder to hip and waist to hip ratios. Evolution and Human Behavior, 24 (3), 173–178.

35   Honekopp, J, U Rudolph, L Beier, a Liebert, and C Muller. "Physical attractiveness of face and body as indicators of physical fitness in men." Evolution and Human Behavior 28, no. 2 (March 2007): 106-111.

attractive when tempered by a touch of "breathiness," suggesting the speaker had a low level of aggression despite his large size.'[36]

Movement: There is even evidence to show that a man's dance moves can attract women! One study identified specific movements within men's dance that affected onlooking women's perceptions of the men's dancing ability, and which are thought to act as signals of male health, vigor or strength.

Another study found that people with more symmetrical bodies are likely to be more proficient dancers. This could mean that a man's dancing skills are a way of signaling his physical fitness.

Other attractive elements: Male attractiveness to heterosexual females is not all about looks, however. There is evidence that women also look for behavioral characteristics that signal a man's ability to provide and protect.

BODY MASS ISSUES

One problem arises when people equate body image with self-image. When people view themselves as being worthy only if they look attractive, problems such as eating disorders arise. Eating disorders can stem from low self-esteem, and from the gap between the cultural ideal of what we are told we should look like and the actuality of how we really look. 'If Marilyn Monroe walked into Weight Watchers today, no one would bat an eye. They'd sign her up.'[37]

---

36   *Human Vocal Attractiveness as Signaled by Body Size Projection. Yi Xu mail, Albert Lee, Wing-Li Wu, Xuan Liu, Peter Birkholz. Published: April 24, 2013. DOI: 10.1371/journal.pone.0062397*
37   *Emily Kravinky, medical director at the Renfrew Center in Philadelphia, a treatment center for women with eating disorders.*

CHANGING YOUR BODY SHAPE

Throughout history, human beings have resorted to 'foundation garments' to change their perceived body shape. Corsets—for both men and women—are among the most famous of these body-augmenting garments. Bustles, stomachers, codpieces, padded brassieres or chest flatteners, cage crinolines, high heels and girdles all pushed and pulled and pinched people into the body shape that was considered ideal at the time.

In Western societies, it was only around the 1960s that women stopped wearing foundation garments as a means of body-shaping. This was due to massive social changes, including feminism and a fashion for more revealing garments. Now that clothes were skimpier, elastic girdles could not be as easily hidden. No longer did women submit to the confinement of tight-fitting undergarments. The benefit to women's health was enormous, but the trend also had its downside. Society demanded that instead of shaping their newly-liberated bodies with underwear, women had to shape them with diet and exercise. The number of people with eating disorders skyrocketed, and the demand for cosmetic surgery exploded.

Some people are dissatisfied with one or more aspects of the way their body looks. However, all bodies are different, and all are beautiful in their own way.

BODY ISSUES: SIGNS OF AGING

Cellulite
The aging process of the collagen and elastic fibers causes the skin's dermis (the middle layer) to become looser and less structured. This allows for more fat cells to protrude into the dermis area, accentuating the appearance of cellulite. Learn more about cellulite on page 36.

Fatty pockets and lumps
Sometimes localized 'fat pockets' form on your stomach, hips, thighs or bottom, showing up as lumps and bumps. It's common to want to get rid of them through spot reduction. Although it's not possible to target weight loss toward specific fat pockets, you can minimize their appearance by losing weight all over. The combination of exercise and a reduced-calorie diet can help you achieve this.

Sagging breasts
Over time, our skin loses elasticity. Women's breasts may sag and droop. To learn more, visit the section on cosmetic surgery under 'Bodysculpt Therapy,' page 68.

Urinary incontinence
Urinary incontinence can affect both males and females. While it is not strictly a cosmetic issue we are including it here because it can be a distressing problem. In the past it could only be addressed with surgery. Urinary incontinence can now be treated with non-invasive laser techniques. The laser used is an Erbium Yag 2940nm, which tightens and lifts the pelvic floor. This laser has been widely employed for facial skin resurfacing and has been shown to be safe and effective.

Wrinkled knees and elbows

Lax skin around the joints creates wrinkles. Dry, flaky patches may also appear. Soothe dry skin with moisturizer containing ammonium lactate or urea—both of these help moisture penetrate the skin. Exfoliate affected areas with a gentle scrub, polish or brush. Learn more about these skin treatments in the companion volume *Ultimate Beauty 1: Face and Skin.*

There is a surgical procedure called a 'knee lift'; there is also a non-invasive 'knee lift' procedure using a combination of infrared light, vacuum and radio frequency. Learn more by reading the section on Knee Lift, page 80.

If dry, saggy elbows are your concern, consider skin-tightening injections.

Varicose and spider veins

As people age, unsightly veins may show through the skin–usually on the face or the legs. There is more information about therapies for varicose and spider veins in the other book in this series: *Ultimate Beauty 1: Face and Skin.*

Skin discoloration

Brownish marks such as 'liver spots' start to appear on our skin as we grow older. Many of these discolored patches are caused by sun damage. Laser skin resurfacing and chemical peels are two of the many possible treatment solutions. Photodynamic therapy, too, can both fade age spots and stimulate collagen production. Keep hands and face well-hydrated.

Always apply sunscreen when heading outdoors – especially on the face, neck and backs of the hands, to prevent further sun damage.

Learn more about therapies for skin discoloration in the section on 'Skin Pigmentation' in the companion book in this series: 'Ultimate Beauty 1: Face and Skin

Snoring

Snoring can be thought of as a cosmetic issue because it deprives people of sleep – and a good night's sleep is essential to our well-being and appearance!

In studies, 'The faces of sleep deprived individuals were perceived as having more hanging eyelids, redder eyes, more swollen eyes, darker circles under the eyes, paler skin, more wrinkles/fine lines, and more droopy corners of the mouth... In addition, sleep-deprived individuals looked sadder than after normal sleep, and sadness was related to looking fatigued.' [38]

According to a study published by the doctors at Dental Sleep and TMD Center of Illinois on May 21, 2014: 'Sleep affects beauty. For quite some time, science has measured that "deep, tired look" of patients who suffer with sleep disturbances. Studies show that patients who resolve their sleep issues often enjoy scientifically-measured improvements in their facial skin. Less redness and forehead puffiness are just two of the noticeable and measurable improvements that can result with improved sleep. In addition, observers who viewed photos of sleep apnea patients after successful treatment often cited these patients as being more attractive, youthful and alert.'

Erbium lasers can provide non-invasive, safe and effective relief from snoring. Some brand names of laser snoring therapies include SleepTight® and NightLase™

---

38   Sundelin T; Lekander M; Kecklund G; Van Someren EJW; Olsson A; Axelsson J. Cues of fatigue: effects of sleep deprivation on facial appearance. SLEEP 2013;36(9):1355-1360.

Thinning hair

Low Level Laser Therapy, also called red light therapy, cold laser, soft laser, biostimulation and photobiomodulation, can be useful in treating hair loss. Learn more in the section on baldness, page 53.

BODY ISSUES: BODY FAT

Why we need body fat

Body fat is vital for the maintenance of life and reproductive functions. Women need more body fat than men, due to the requirements of childbearing and breastfeeding.

'Body fat percentage' is a measure of a person's relative body composition in which height or weight is irrelevant. The commonly used body mass index (BMI) compares the adiposity (amount of fat) of individuals of different heights and weights.

While a person's BMI generally increases as their body's fat content increases, it is not really an accurate indicator of body fat. For example, people with more muscle mass or bigger bones will have higher BMIs.

Obesity, the condition of being excessively fat or overweight, is a growing health problem around the world. Many cosmetic treatments are being offered to help those who are unable to lose weight using diet and exercise.

Even people who are not obese may worry if they carry unsightly pockets of body fat that cause lumps and bulges.

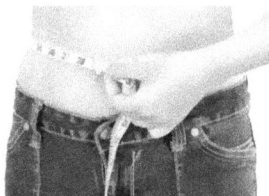

Cosmetic procedures for removing excess body fat include:

- Acoustic wave therapy
- Body contouring surgery
- Body wraps
- Combination of rollers plus vacuuming
- Fat freezing
- Fat transfer
- Laser cellulite/fat removal
- Lipodissolve
- Liposuction
- Mesotherapy injections
- Microcurrent
- Radiofrequency
- Ultrasound
- Vacuum fat removal
- Vaser

Tips for getting rid of excess body fat naturally:

- Engage in regular cardio-vascular stimulating activities such as brisk walking, jogging, cycling, dancing and/or swimming.
- Lift weights.
- Drink more water.
- Consume fewer calories than you burn.
- Eat nutritious foods.
- Reduce your intake of sugar.
- Reduce your intake of starchy carbohydrates, such as those found in bread, cakes, potatoes, pasta.
- Eat a full, balanced breakfast.
- Avoid drastic calorie reductions, as this can tip your body into 'starvation mode', which makes it harder to lose fat.

BODY ISSUES: FAT POCKETS

Fat accumulates in certain areas of the body based on many factors including hereditary factors, your sex, age and body weight. Localized fat or 'fat pockets', showing up as lumps and bumps, may form on your stomach, hips, thighs, back, knees or buttocks.

Fat pockets on non-obese people

Even people who are not obese may wish to be rid of unsightly pockets of body fat that cause lumps and bulges.

When unwanted fat pockets form it is not possible to get rid of them by way of 'spot reduction'. Targeting weight loss toward specific fat pockets simply does not work. You can only get rid of them by:

- Surgical cosmetic treatments
- Non-surgical or minimally invasive cosmetic treatments
- Losing weight all over (see our tips for getting rid of excess body fat naturally)

Surgical cosmetic treatments for fat pockets include:

- Body contouring surgery
- Fat transfer
- Liposuction

Minimally invasive[39] treatments for fat pockets include:

- Lipodissolve
- Mesotherapy injections

---

39   'Minimally invasive': injections or cannulas are involved.

Non-surgical treatments for fat pockets include:

- Acoustic wave therapy
- Body wraps
- Fat freezing
- Laser
- Microcurrent treatments
- Radiofrequency treatments
- Ultrasound treatments

BODY ISSUES: CELLULITE

Fat deposits often become trapped and squeezed between the stiffened fibrous bands that connect the skin's tissues, leading to the dreaded puckered effect on upper and outer thighs and buttocks, and also the stomach and arms. This is what is called 'cellulite'. The phenomenon is largely unrelated to weight, because even slim supermodels can have it.

Less than five per cent of men suffer from cellulite. Men tend to have large, loose, unconnected fat cells that don't have a lot of blood supply, and don't develop the fibrous tissues.

The Cellulite Grading System

The most common cellulite grading system is referred to as the Nurenberg scale, named after the German physician who invented it in 1972.

- Grade 1 means there is no obvious cellulite when a person is standing, but if she pinches the skin on the thighs there will be an orange-peel appearance.

- Grades 2 and 3 each have three variants – mild, moderate and severe – meaning that there are actually seven levels of cellulite, in all.

- Grade 2 refers to cellulite that's visible while standing and sitting, and grade 3 to that which is extremely visible while standing, sitting or lying down.

Cellulite treatments include:
- Acoustic wave therapy
- Cellulaze®
- Combination treatments
- Endermologie®
- Hypoxi®
- Laser cellulite treatments
- Liopdissolve
- Mesotherapy
- Radiofrequency (RF) cellulite treatments
- Subcision surgery
- Ultrasound cellulite treatments

For information on treatments for cellulite, visit our Cellulite Reduction section, page 109.

BODY ISSUES: SAGGING BODY SKIN

Collagen and elastin are two substances within your skin that help to keep its structure firm. However, skin on the face and/or body may start to loosen and sag, due to a number of possible causes.

These include:

Age. With the passing years, our skin's collagen and elastin production naturally declines. The skin loses its natural elasticity.

Lifestyle. Smoking and sun exposure can 'prematurely age' your skin and cause sagging. Fine lines and wrinkles can appear in dry, sun damaged, dry skin. Over time, these can lead to sagginess.

Weight Loss. Extreme or rapid weight loss may also give you saggy skin. Skin that sags as a result of weight loss may become firmer if you practice moisturizing and exfoliating regimens regularly over one to two years.

Genetics. Your genetic heritage may predispose the skin to sag on certain parts of your body.

Lack of muscle tone. The underlying muscles that support your skin gradually weaken as you age. As a result, fat may accumulate in 'baggy' areas. When people lose weight primarily by dieting, without exercising, their skin may sag.

Fluid retention. This can puff up the tissues of the skin, stretching them and causing the formation of saggy skin.

Slower skin recycling. As we age, our skin gradually loses its ability to shed dead skin cells. This, too, can contribute to skin-sag.

COSMETIC PROCEDURES TO TIGHTEN SAGGING BODY SKIN:

Cosmetic surgeons can actually cut off and remove a patient's sagging body skin. This gives the appearance of tighter skin overall. Other therapies which help to tighten sagging body skin are generally non-invasive or minimally-invasive. They include:

- Acoustic wave therapy
- Chemical peels
- Dermabrasion
- Dermal fillers
- Laser skin resurfacing
- Laser skin tightening treatments
- Mesotherapy
- Radiofrequency
- Skin tightening injections
- Ultrasound

NATURAL WAYS TO TIGHTEN SAGGING BODY SKIN:

Exercise. Weight training can condition, strengthen and tone the muscles underlying your skin. Firmer muscles supporting the skin may make it look less saggy.

Exfoliate. Exfoliate your skin to scrub away dead skin cells, promote regeneration of new skin and encourage healthy circulation.

Moisturize. Moisturize your skin to improve and prevent sagging. Staying hydrated and moisturizing your skin helps prevent fluid retention and keeps your skin cells plump and firm. Hyaluronic acid skin-care products can help to restore the skin's moisture.

Drink water. When you drink plenty of water it is like using a moisturizer, but from the inside. By adding moisture to your skin you are making the cells fuller and softer. If the cells are dry, then drinking water will plump them up.

Use sunscreen. Protect your skin from the sun by applying sunscreen before going outdoors. This won't firm up your skin but it will stop it from losing even more elasticity.

Eat well.
A diet rich in skin-friendly vitamins and minerals, especially zinc and selenium, can help preserve your skin's existing elasticity.

Skin creams. There are various topical skin creams on the market, whose manufacturers claim that their use can actually induce collagen and elastin production in the skin, thus increasing elasticity. Some of their ingredients include:

- aloe vera extract
- copper peptides
- pentapeptides
- yeast extract
- soy protein
- pomegranate

Aloe vera: The University of Maryland Medical Center reports that 'Aloe, ginger, grape seed extract, and coral extracts contain antioxidants and are promoted as being healthy for the skin. However, evidence of their effects on wrinkles is weak.'

Copper peptides: Inside our bodies, together with vitamin C and the mineral zinc, copper helps to develop elastin, the fibers that support skin structure from beneath.

Doctors warn that consuming copper supplements can be dangerous; topical applications of copper-rich creams, on the other hand, are not associated with the same risks.

Studies presented at the American Academy of Dermatology Annual Meeting in 2002 showed that a cream containing copper peptides could noticeably firm the skin and help restore some thickness and elasticity.

The research, conducted at the University of Pennsylvania, concluded that the a cream gave rapid, visual overall improvements in skin texture, clarity, fine lines, wrinkling, and overall sun damage.

Pentapeptides: An investigation by the United Kingdom's Advertising Standards Authority (ASA) reported that 'scientific evidence does not show that pentapeptides are effective at reducing the appearance of lines and wrinkles.'

Yeast extract: It is possible that yeast extract might have some benefits for the skin, however its effects have not yet been thoroughly explored.

Soy protein and pomegranate: 'Pomegranate and soy extracts may help rejuvenate aging skin', according to the University of Maryland Medical Center.

Part 2:
Teeth Issues

TEETH ISSUES

WHAT MAKES TEETH ATTRACTIVE?

Teeth that are white and evenly spaced make people appear more attractive. Studies have suggested that this is because teeth are a sign of health and reproductive fitness. [40]

Researchers showed photos of male and female models to men and women. In some of the photos, the researchers had digitally altered the color and spacing of the teeth. Models who showed even, white teeth were rated as attractive, while those same models with discolored, and/or uneven teeth were rated as less attractive.

Yellow or widely-spaced teeth were particularly unpopular. The condition of women's teeth had a particularly potent effect on both the men looking at the photos and the women. The researchers explained this by saying, 'Males are thinking about attraction and females are in competition with each other.'

In the study, the brilliant white teeth which are the result of cosmetic whitening processes were not considered any more attractive than evenly spaced, evenly colored teeth of a more natural shade.

As we get older, our teeth get darker. Tooth enamel wears away over time. It can also become stained. The condition of a woman's teeth can not only signify her age, however; it can also provide evidence of childhood illnesses, the food she eats and some genetic disorders.

40   Evidence to Suggest That Teeth Act as Human Ornament Displays Signaling Mate Quality. Colin A. Hendrie mail, Gayle Brewer. PLoS ONE Published: July 31, 2012. DOI: 10.1371/journal.pone.0042178

Cosmetic issues with teeth, such as discoloration and unevenness, can be treated with laser, light therapies, orthodontics, medications and topical preparations.

DISCOLORED TEETH

Teeth may become discolored with extrinsic stains (superficial stains found on the surface of the tooth) or intrinsic stains (stains formed deep within the tooth). Tooth discoloration can happen for the following reasons:

- Food and drink, especially the consumption of tea, coffee, red wine and/or soft drinks over a prolonged period. These cause extrinsic stains.
- Smoking (extrinsic stains).
- Tooth injury (intrinsic stains).
- Age. No matter how well you clean your teeth, they will eventually become duller as you age. This is due to intrinsic staining.

See page 122 for methods of teeth whitening.

OTHER TEETH ISSUES

Other teeth and mouth problems can include misshapen or crooked teeth, missing teeth, misshapen gums and uneven gum lines.

For information on ways to deal with these issues, read "Teeth Therapy" on page 121

Part 3:
Hair Issues

HAIR ISSUES

WHAT MAKES HEAD-HAIR ATTRACTIVE?

People of different cultures and different historical periods have viewed the hair that grows from the scalp in a wide range of ways. Hairstyles and fashions in hair colors come and go. The arrangement of one's hair is often used to indicate one's personal beliefs, age, sex, religion or social position.[41]

Hair color

It is often claimed that men prefer blond women. 'Flaxen' is the hair-color of beautiful princesses in fairytales, and a multitude of Hollywood actresses have been blond. Ten years after Charles Darwin published 'On the Origin of Species' in 1859, the great man began studying the sexual selection of blond hair in women, in readiness for his book 'The Descent of Man and Selection in Relation to Sex', which was later published in 1871. He was, however, unable to find enough data to support his theory that blond hair is sexually selected and abandoned his research.

Blond hair is more common during youth. The blond locks of children generally darken as they grow older, so if males really do prefer blond women, it might be because (prior to the ready availability of hydrogen peroxide), blond hair in females could be interpreted as a sign of youth, and thus reproductive fitness.

---

41   Sherrow, Victoria (2006). Encyclopedia of Hair: A Cultural History. 88 Post Road West, Westport, CT: Greenwood Press. p. iv. ISBN 0-313-33145-6.

Blondness is not always perceived as desirable. In central Africa, for example, the birth of an albino baby arouses superstitious fear that can lead to infanticide.

More girls are born blond than boys. One study found that females whose hair remains naturally blond into adulthood are generally physically fitter.[42]

Caucasian blondes generally have slightly higher estrogen levels than brunettes. They also tend to have other characteristics that indicate low levels of testosterone and are considered attractive by males, such as finer facial features, smaller noses and jaws, pointed chins, narrow shoulders, evenly-textured skin and sparse body hair, and childlike behavior such as liveliness and playfulness.[43]

Blond hair in males is no indicator of estrogen levels as it is in females; nor is it a sign of fitness as it is in females. Furthermore, unlike men, women do not base their choice of mate on physical appearance to the degree that men do. This might explain why blondness, if it is an attractive trait, is generally judged to be desirable in women.

Hair abundance

Abundant scalp hair can be viewed in a variety of ways, according to one's cultural background.

'In Australia, balding Aranda Aborigines once wore wigs made of emu feathers. Likewise, the Azande in Sudan wore wigs made of sponge. To grow long hair among the Ashanti in Nigeria made one suspect of contemplating murder,

---

42   Ridley, M (1993) The Red Queen: Sex and the Evolution of Human Nature. Penguin.

43   Grammer, K, Thornhill, R et al (2003) Darwinian aesthetics: sexual selection and the biology of beauty. Biological Reviews; 78(3): 385-407.

while in Brazil the Bororo people cut their hair as a sign of mourning.'[44]

In most cultures, short hair signals restraint and discipline. Generally, the hair of prisoners, soldiers, and monks is short. Long hair tends to signify freedom and individualism. The hippies of the 1960s and the cavalier royalists of the 17th century wore their hair long, in contrast to their opposites, the 'skinheads' and the 'roundheads'.

Human hair chiefly grows from the scalp, but may appear anywhere else on the body, especially the eyebrows, underarms and pubic region. Hair grows from beneath the skin. The living parts of hair lie beneath the skin, while the visible hair shaft (the cuticle) has no living processes. Damage to the hair shaft cannot be repaired by biological processes such as nutrition, though much can be done to help the cuticle remain intact.

Cosmetic hair issues can include unwanted body hair, thinning scalp hair, patchy baldness, pattern balding, loss of eyelashes and thinning of eyebrows.

HAIR'S STRUCTURE

Hair is made up of two structures – the follicle and the hair shaft. At the base of the follicle is a projection called a papilla and it contains capillaries, or tiny blood vessels, that feed the cells. The living part of the hair is the bottom part surrounding the papilla. It's called the bulb. The bulb is the

---

44   *The Enigma of Beauty. Written by Cathy Newman. National Geographic magazine*

only part fed by the capillaries. The cells in the bulb divide every 23 to 72 hours, faster than any other cells in the body.

The follicle is surrounded by two sheaths – an inner and outer sheath. These sheaths protect and mold the growing hair shaft. The inner sheath follows the hair shaft down into the skin and ends underneath the opening of a sebaceous (oil) gland. The sebaceous gland is important because it produces sebum, which is a natural conditioner. After we reach puberty our bodies produce more sebum. Women's sebum production decreases throughout their lives. The production also decreases in men, but not as much as in women.

The hair shaft is made up of dead, hard protein called keratin in three layers. The inner layer is called the medulla. The next layer is the cortex and it makes up the majority of the hair shaft. The outer layer is the cuticle. Most hair conditioning products attempt to affect the cuticle. There are pigment cells that are distributed throughout the cortex and medulla giving the hair its color.

HAIR'S GROWTH CYCLE

Hair on the scalp grows about 0.3—0.4 millimeters per day, or about 6 inches per year. Human hair growth and loss is haphazard and not seasonal or cyclic. At any given time, a random number of hairs will be in various stages of growth and shedding.

There are three stages of hair growth: catagen, telogen, and anagen.

Catagen – The catagen phase is a transitional stage and 3% of all hairs are in this phase at any time. This phase lasts for about 2—3 weeks. During this time growth stops and the outer root sheath shrinks and attaches to the root of the hair. This is the formation of what is known as a club hair.

Telogen – Telogen is the resting phase and accounts for 10—15% of all hairs. This phase lasts for about 100 days for hairs on the scalp and much longer for hairs on the eyebrow, eyelash, arm and leg. During this phase the hair follicle is completely at rest and the club hair is completely formed. If you pull out a hair that is in the telogen phase, you will notice at its root a tiny clump of hard, dry, whitish material. Normally we shed around 25—100 telogen hairs every day.

Anagen – Anagen is the active phase of hair growth, during which the cells in the root of the hair are dividing rapidly. When a new hair is formed it pushes the club hair up the follicle and eventually out through the skin. During this phase the hair grows about 1 cm (approximately ½ inch) every 28 days.

Scalp hair remains in this active phase for 2—6 years. It is hard for some people to grow their hair beyond a certain length because their anagen phase is short. Conversely, people who are able to grow their hair long have a prolonged anagen phase.

The reason why the hairs on the eyebrows, eyelashes, arms and legs are shorter than the hair on the head is because they have a very short active growth phase; around 30—45 days.

CURLY OR STRAIGHT, SHINY OR DULL?

The amount of natural curl a hair possesses is determined by its cross-sectional shape.

The more circular the shaft is, the straighter it is. The more elliptical the shaft is, the curlier or kinkier the hair.

The cross-sectional shape also determines the amount of shine the hair has. Straighter hair is shinier because sebum from the sebaceous gland can travel down the hair more easily.

The kinkier the hair, the more difficulty the sebum has traveling down the hair, therefore the more dry or dull the hair looks.

HAIR ISSUES: BALDNESS

There are several types of baldness, including the following:

PATTERN BALDING

Pattern balding is related to your genes and sex hormones. Male pattern baldness (androgenic alopecia) usually follows a pattern of receding hairline and hair thinning on the crown, and is caused by hormones and genetic predisposition.

The reason for the less common female pattern baldness (which is also called 'androgenic alopecia') is not well understood, but may be related to aging, changes in the levels of androgens (male hormones) after menopause, and family history of male or female pattern baldness.

PATCHY BALDNESS

Patchy baldness is otherwise known as alopecia areata. It is a common autoimmune disease that can affect any hair-bearing area of the body, and its cause is not fully understood.

This type of baldness can appear as a single, well defined patch of hair loss, loss of eyelashes or eyebrows, many patches, or extensive hair loss in the form of total loss of scalp hair (alopecia totalis) or loss of entire scalp and body hair (alopecia universalis). Patients with extensive baldness may choose to wear scalp prostheses, such as wigs or hairpieces.

COMPLETE BALDNESS

Complete loss of hair on the scalp is known as alopecia areata totalis. Alopecia acreata universalis is the rarest form of alopecia areata and involves the loss of all body hair including eyelashes, underarms and eyebrows.

TEMPORARY OR REVERSIBLE HAIR LOSS

Some factors that can cause temporary or reversible hair loss include pregnancy, physical trauma, emotional stress, illness, too much vitamin A, a severely protein-deficient diet, some contraceptives, anemia, hypothyroidism, vitamin B deficiency, chemotherapy, sudden weight loss, polycystic ovary syndrome, overstyling, trichotillomania, antidepressants, anabolic steroids, blood thinners and other medications.

HAIR ISSUES: UNWANTED BODY HAIR

Unwanted body hair refers to hair growing in socially unacceptable or personally unacceptable body areas, or even hair growing in esthetically unpleasing ways, such as elongated and wiry eyebrow hairs.

Unwanted hair may appear as nostril or ear hair in older men, facial hair in older women or women with hirsutism, eyebrows growing in an undesirable shape or position, or pubic, chest, back or underarm hair that has fallen out of vogue. In fact, hair anywhere at all on the body can be the subject of fluctuations in fashion.

Unwanted body hair on women

It is estimated that approximately 40% of women have some measure of unwanted facial hair.[45]

A condition called 'facial hirsutism' occurs in between 5—15% of all women from all ethnic backgrounds.

Hirsutism is generally caused by an adrenal, ovarian, or central endocrine imbalance. Women afflicted with facial hirsutism usually suffer from a great deal of personal distress, such as depression and anxiety, and often experience difficulty in social situations.

The normal amount of facial and body hair for women varies. In general, women only have fine hair, sometimes called 'peach fuzz', growing above the upper lip and along the jaw and chin; also in the armpits, one the pubic area and on the legs. Women with hirsutism may have coarse, dark hairs in these areas, as well as on the back, chest and abdomen.

---

45   Blume-Peytavi U, Gieler U, Hoffmann R, Shapiro J,. "Unwanted Facial Hair: Affects, Effects and Solutions. Dermatology. 2007; 215(2): 139-46".

One cause of hirsutism is a hormonal condition called polycystic ovarian syndrome (PCOS).

Unwanted body hair on men

Fashion in men's body hair is ever-changing. Depending on the latest trend, men may wish to rid themselves of hair on their face, neck, chest, back, pubic area, legs, arms ... indeed, just about anywhere on the body, including the head.

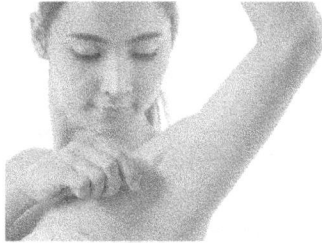

HAIR ISSUES: THE HAIR ON THE HEAD

The appearance of the hair on your head has several components of its own:

- Texture—whether the hairs are fine or coarse, smooth or rough, curly or straight.
- Color—natural hair colors range from jet black through brown and auburn to blond, gray and white. Hair dyes have an almost limitless range of colors.
- Shape—by this we mean the overall shape of your hairstyle. It may be upstanding, wide, long, short, shaved, voluminous etc.
- Style—for example page-boy, mullet beehive, bouffant, tousled, quiffed, crimped, permed.

- Balance—oily, normal or dry.
- Condition—healthy or damaged by sun, ill-health, chemicals etc.
- Abundance—plentiful, thick hair or sparse hair.

Any of these components can be treated. We discuss head-hair treatments later in this book, page 129.

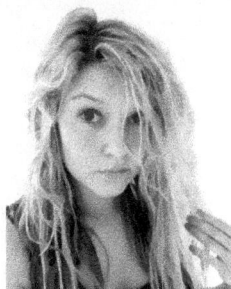

HAIR ISSUES: EYEBROWS AND EYELASHES

Eyebrow issues may include too much or too little hair or no hair at all, asymmetry of the eyebrow shape or position, unwanted eyebrow shape or position, undesirable color, texture or length of the eyebrow hairs,

Many therapies exist for maintaining or recreating the shape and position of the eyebrows. These include plucking, waxing, threading, electrolysis, cosmetic tattooing, eyebrow transplant and dyeing.

Eyelashes can enhance the look of the eyes and the face. Problems with the appearance of the eyelashes can include lack of eyelashes altogether, sparse lashes, over-short lashes, over-long lashes or lashes that are an unwanted color. These issues can generally be addressed with treatments such as prosthetics, cosmetic tattooing and makeup.

Since eyebrows and eyelashes are integral to the overall look of the face, we do not discuss their treatments here; instead they are included in our sequel book '*Ultimate Beauty 1: Face and Skin.*

Part 4:
Body Reshaping

BODY RESHAPING

THE FASHION HISTORY OF BODY SHAPE

Throughout human history (and probably pre-history as well), the 'ideal' body shape for men and women has been subject to the whims of fashion. The idea of what is beautiful will continue to change as the years roll by.

Clothing can alter the body's appearance by boosting it, constricting it, lengthening or shortening it (as with high-heeled shoes), changing the apparent proportions, or creating an illusion by the skillfull use of color and design.

Judging by statues that were created by the Greeks and Romans in ancient times, the ideal young man was lightly muscled, with low body fat. The statues show no evidence of the bulging veins of striations or veins that would appear if they were body builders. They look like men who keep fit by way of normal exercise. Michelangelo's statue of David too, crafted during the Renaissance, shows a fit young man, well-muscled and quite lean.

Paintings created during the Renaissance depict voluptuous women. These artists' models were fêted for their full, curvaceous figures. By the standards of 21st century western societies, they would be considered overweight.

Henry VIII, in the 16th century, wore corsets beneath his clothes to encompass his corpulent body—as did other men of the period. Men also favored codpieces; padded, oversized and reinforced pouches worn at the crotch, to accentuate their manly genital area. Henry showed off his shapely legs, of which he was proud, by wearing tight-fitting hose, often in garish colors.

Panniers or side hoops were undergarments worn by upper class European women during the 17th and 18th centuries. They served to extend the width of the skirts at the sides, while leaving the front and back comparatively flat. The idea was to provide a panel of fabric on which sumptuous embellishments could be displayed; it also made women's hips look inordinately wide and their waists look relatively small.

During the Victorian era the ideal female had an extremely narrow waist. To achieve this look, women wore corsets to pull in their bodies at the waistline. Sometimes these undergarments were laced so tightly that the wearers could hardly breathe. There are records of ribcages breaking under the strain—even of death caused by broken ribs puncturing internal organs.

At the same time, the shape and prominence of the buttocks was enhanced by the attachment of bustles and layered petticoats.

The 1920s were years in which women tried to hide their curves. Some would even bind their chests with lengths of fabric to make themselves look boyish or androgynous. They swapped waist-cinching corsets for webbed elastic girdles, which made the abdomen appear flat. The straight-up-and-down 'flapper' look was in huge contrast to the bosomy, 'busty', extravagantly curved female figure of the Victorian era.

During the 1930s and 1940s shoulder-pads were all the rage in women's and men's costume, giving the illusion of broad shoulders. Women were still wearing 'foundation garments' at this time, to pinch in their waists. Padded bras were also introduced and as the 1950s advanced, women's skirts flared wider. By the middle of the 20th century, the hourglass figure was back.

What about men? If you watch old movies about Superman, Batman and Tarzan, where the physiques of the heroes were revealed by tight-fitting or sparse clothing, you will notice a distinct difference between them and the screen heroes of the 21st century. While all of the actors who played these classic roles are tall and broad-shouldered, their bodies are what might now be deemed 'soft and flabby'.

Up to the 1960s women could still alter the appearance of their body shape by using undergarments such as corsets and girdles. With the new revealing clothes, however, if they wanted to conform to the fashionable ideal, they had to change their actual bodies.

Emulating the famous, stick-thin models of the 1960s such as Twiggy, many women's lives became dominated by the quest for weight loss. Hippie girls, despite their more casual, flowing garments, were affected by the drive to be slim, no less than mini-skirted Twiggy-copiers.

The quest for feminine thinness now had a firm grip on western society. It continued throughout the 1970s, the big-haired, broad-shouldered, aerobics-obsessed 1980s and the grungy, minimalist 1990s.

In fact, it was in the mid-1990s that the term 'heroin chic' was coined, to describe a waif-like, emaciated look characterized by pale skin and dark circles underneath the eyes. The unhealthy appearance of a drug addict had become a sought-after look.

As we travel further into the 21st century, western society still expects women to aspire to an impossibly thin body shape.

Meanwhile, practically every study of male body shape and attractiveness confirms that the masculine, V-shaped, athletic physique is most appealing. Across cultures, the ideal man's body shape appears to be wide-shouldered, long-torsoed, long-legged, tall, slim-waisted, slim-hipped, muscular and youthful, with shapely buttocks.

COLLAGEN AND ELASTIN

When discussing sagging skin on the body, it is important to know something about the roles played by collagen and elastin. The following information is quoted from the companion volume, '*Ultimate Beauty 1: Face and Skin.*

'Collagen and elastin are two biological substances that occur naturally in our skin. Together they are responsible for the skin's strength, firmness, and shape.

Collagen

'"Collagen" is the term for a group of proteins that mostly occur in our connective or 'fibrous' tissues. They are the most common proteins in the human body, comprising around 30% of total protein content.

'Connective or 'fibrous' tissues support and/or connect other forms of tissues or body organs. Their role is to strengthen the other tissues and support their shape. Some examples of connective tissues include cartilage, fat and tendons. Collagen is abundant in our skin, but is also part of our ligaments, blood vessels, bones, and eyes.

Elastin

'Like collagen, elastin is a protein that is located in connective tissues. It is, however, a different type of protein. Elastin is elastic; that is, it enables the body's tissues to 'snap back' to their original shape after they have been contracted or stretched. An example of skin stretching occurs when we smile, or make any other facial expression. Elastin can be compared to a rubber band.

'Our artery walls, lungs, intestines and skin all contain elastin. All these tissues need to be able to expand and contract to keep us healthy. When young skin containing abundant elastin is pinched or pulled, it resumes its normal shape when released. Elastin is responsible for this.

The Collagen-Elastin Combination

'Collagen is composed of very strong fibers with exceptional tensile strength. These fibers provide the foundation to anchor the skin's outer layer. Elastin, despite being essential for skin function, is not as abundant in the skin as collagen. It forms an elastic network between the collagen fibers. It could be said that collagen is for skin structure while elastin is for skin "bounce".

'These two proteins are important in skin care because their actions combine to give skin its shape and firmness. Collagen, the basic supporting structure, provides density, compactness and volume, while elastin lets stretched skin return to the shape collagen gives it.

Collagen and Elastin Deficiency

'The process of aging depletes the skin of these two important proteins. In young skin, collagen and elastin are abundant. Skin looks smooth and taut. As years go by, the body's production of collagen and elastin decreases. Sun damage, pollution and other factors also contribute to the breaking down of the skin's connective fibers. The skin becomes thinner and even more vulnerable to sun damage and other environmental aggravations.

'When skin is deficient in collagen and elastin it sags and wrinkles. The elastin in aging skin begins to lose its ability to snap back, just as a rubber band that is continually stretched will, over time, lose its resilience. When this happens, our skin sags. Usually we notice this most around the eyes, jaw line, and neck.'

COSMETIC BODY RESHAPING METHODS

Body reshaping, also known as 'bodysculpting or 'bodysculpt therapy', involves changing muscle density, gaining, losing, moving or removing fat, surgically altering body parts or adding implants to achieve a desired body shape.

Reshaping the body (and face) can be done in numerous ways. The most natural way is to exercise and eat well. Weight-lifting exercises can increase muscle mass, adding definition to the body and limbs, and giving support to sagging skin. Eating well to lose fat can get rid of unsightly body bulges and double chins.

①Surgical therapies for body reshaping include:

- Arm lift (brachioplasty)
- Breast augmentation (augmentation mammoplasty)
- Breast lift (mastopexy)
- Brow lift (forehead lift)
- Buttock implant
- Buttock lift
- Cellulite subcission surgery
- Fat transfer
- Knee lift
- Liposuction
- Lower body lift
- Skin tightening surgery
- Thigh lift
- Tummy tuck (abdominoplasty)

②Minimally invasive therapies for body reshaping include:

- Cellulaze®
- Dermal fillers
- Fat freezing
- Laser liposuction
- Laser skin tightening
- Lipodissolve
- Liposuction
- Mesotherapy
- Microcurrent skin tightening
- Vacuum suction

Non-surgical therapies for body reshaping include:

- Acoustic wave therapy
- Body-shaping undergarments
- Diet and exercise
- Endermologie®
- Fat freezing
- Hypoxi®
- Laser cellulite treatments
- Microcurrent therapy
- Radiofrequency fat disruption
- Ultrasound therapy

FRUGAL BODY RESHAPING

- Lose fat by eating, in moderation, a wide range of nutritious, unprocessed foods.
- Exercise regularly, to build muscle.
- Wear body-shaping foundation garments or flattering clothes.
- Accept your appearance; consulting a counselor or psychologist may help you conquer your dissatisfaction with your looks, and you might end up being happy with your own, unique beauty.

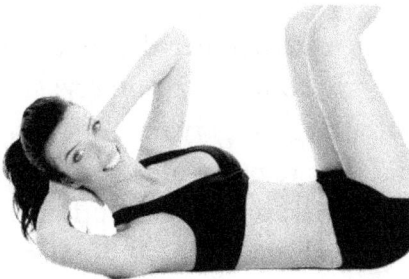

SURGICAL BODY RESHAPING: COSMETIC SURGERY

Cosmetic surgery is an invasive procedure that can be performed on all areas of the head, neck and body.

For information on cosmetic surgery for the face, see the other book in this series – *Ultimate Beauty 1: Face and Skin.*

Body reshaping/contouring is a type of cosmetic surgery whose purpose is to enhance the patient's appearance. It involves the use of a scalpel to cut away extra fat and sagging skin, thus making the body appear slimmer and the skin appear tighter, or the insertion of implants to 'bulk out' certain body areas.

The result is a body with fewer bulges and smoother contours. People sometimes opt for this procedure after they have lost a large amount of weight and their skin has not been able to fully shrink back into place, leaving them with a 'baggy' look. Areas that are often affected by loose, sagging skin include the upper arms, breasts, abdomen, buttocks, groin and thighs.

Usually, patients undergoing body contouring surgery will be placed under a general anesthetic. Surgeons will often perform body contouring in stages. A full 'body overhaul' may take months, or even years, to complete.

It is important to remember the following points if you are considering body contouring surgery:

* Body contouring surgery is not intended to simply remove excess fat. For removal of excess fat pockets, liposuction would be a more appropriate option. If your skin has good elasticity (stretchiness) it will bounce back to tighten

against your remodeled body contours after liposuction. Skin elasticity is more common in younger people. If your skin's elasticity is poor, your doctor might recommend a combination of liposuction and body contouring techniques; ie the surgical removal of the sagging skin left behind after liposuction.

* Before you have any body contouring surgery, your weight should be stable. If you lose weight after surgery, you may end up with loose pockets of skin. On the other hand if you gain weight, your surgically tightened skin will be forced to stretch too far, creating stretch marks and expanding your surgical scars.

* During the body contouring procedure, your surgeon will have to make numerous cuts. Expect some pretty extensive scarring. The surgeon will try to place incisions within natural skin folds and in places where your clothes will hide the scars. Concealing scars is not always possible, however, and some may be visible.

* Stop smoking. Smokers are always at increased risk of surgical complications.

* Even if you are a non-smoker, there can be complications following any form of surgery. Your surgeon will inform you of any risks.

Cosmetic surgery procedures for body reshaping include:

- Arm lift (brachioplasty)
- Breast augmentation (augmentation mammoplasty)
- Breast lift (mastopexy)
- Buttock implant
- Buttock lift
- Cellulite subcission surgery
- Fat transfer
- Knee lift
- Liposuction
- Lower body lift
- Skin tightening surgery
- Thigh lift
- Tummy tuck (abdominoplasty)
- Fat transfer/grafting

When people undergo many or all of these surgeries, it is called a 'body lift'.

SURGICAL BODY RESHAPING: ARM LIFT

Arm lifting surgery is called 'brachioplasty'.

As we age, the skin of the upper arms loses elasticity and becomes more likely to sag. Sagging of the skin on the upper arms can also occur if we lose a lot of weight.

Arm lifting surgery reshapes the underside of the upper arm, so that the arms look slimmer and more toned. The surgeon makes an incision from the armpit down to the elbow, then inserts a thin tube called a cannula into the layers of fat. The excess fat is then vacuumed out, using the process known as liposuction.

The surgeon uses stitches to tighten the muscles underlying the fat, thereby defining the shape of the upper arm. Some of the skin is cut away, then the surgeon closes the incision with more stitches.

The procedure leaves a scar running down the inside of the upper arms. This scar will remain forever, although it may fade significantly as time goes by.

Patients undergoing arm lifts are given a general anesthetic. The procedure can take up to three hours.

All surgery carries some degree of risk. Ask your surgeon about the risks and potential complications of brachioplasty.

Arm lifts do not guarantee slim, toned arms for the rest of your life. If you later gain, and then lose a significant amount of weight, your stretched skin will sag again.

SURGICAL BODY RESHAPING: BACK LIFT

Back lift surgery is sometimes called a 'bra lift'.

It is used for reshaping the bodies of patients with rolls of fat and sagging skin in the middle, upper and lower back.

In this procedure the surgeon cuts off the excess skin and removes the fat from the upper part of the back, extending into the armpits. This surgery can also be used to pare away the excess skin that extends around the sides of the body if the patient wishes. The surgeon makes an incision into the part of the back which, in women, is usually hidden by a bra, so that the scar will be less visible.

A back lift not only improves the contours of the upper back; it also helps to re-contour the skin on the lower back because there is less fat and skin pressing down on the lower area.

SURGICAL BODY RESHAPING: BREAST AUGMENTATION

BREAST AUGMENTATION - IMPLANTS

'Breast augmentation' is also known as 'augmentation mammoplasty'. These terms refer to the surgical procedure of making the breasts larger (or changing their shape) by means of breast-implants or fat-transfers/grafting.

A breast implant is a prosthesis that consists of a flexible sac or shell made of solid silicone. This sac is filled with a gel-like or fluid material, usually silicone or saline (salt water).

Silicone-filled Implants

Up till 1994 silicone-filled breast implants contained liquid silicone. The major drawback of this was that sometimes the sacs leaked, allowing silicone to enter the body and create significant health problems. Those implants are no longer manufactured. Instead, silicone-filled implants now contain a cohesive gel that does not leak into the surrounding breast tissue if the sac develops a puncture. The newer sacs are also less likely to rupture. Because silicone gel implants cannot leak, they are the most popular with both surgeons and patients. Also, silicone gel feels and looks more natural and ripples less than saline.

Disadvantages of silicone-filled implants include the potential for 'capsular contracture' over time. Capsular contracture happens when the body's immune system reacts to foreign materials. It involves the formation of capsules of tightly-woven collagen fibers, as if the immune system is 'cordoning off' the foreign object from the rest of the body. Over the course of a lifetime, silicone implants may begin to look less natural as a 'capsule' of hard flesh forms around them. The collagen-fiber capsule tightens and squeezes the breast implant. This can be very painful, and can distort the shape of the breast.

Saline implants

The surgical incision is smaller with saline-filled implants and larger with those filled with silicone gel. Silicone implants arrive pre-filled, at a pre-set size, and are not adjustable in the operating room. Saline implants on the other hand, are more adjustable, which means that the surgeon can alter the size during surgery; for example, to compensate for any asymmetry in the breasts. The development of hardened scars, over time, is much less common than in patients with silicone gel implants.

Polyurethane coated implants (PCIs)

Polyurethane coated implants or 'porous coated' implants are made of silicone gel coated with polyurethane. The idea is to reduce the chance of capsular contracture by provoking an inflammatory reaction in the body. Such a reaction hinders the formation of fibrous collagen capsules around the implant. The early polyurethane coated implants caused health issues. Contemporary PCIs do not cause those problems; however they are the most difficult implants for surgeons to place into position.

Over the months following the breast augmentation procedure, the coating of the PCIs dissolves in the body. It's true that this does result in a low rate of capsular contracture; however the drawback is that if the implants have to be removed or repositioned for any reason during the period of dissolving, it could be an extremely difficult task.

Shapes of Implants

The two main shapes for breast implants are round and tear-drop.

Round implants are dome-shaped and look like the breasts of a woman who is lying on her back. They keep this 'perky' shape even when the woman stands up—unlike real breasts, whose soft tissue is affected by gravity. These are the most popular implants.

Tear-drop shaped implants (called 'anatomical implants') more closely resemble the shape of a real breast.

Volume and Protrusion

Most women seeking breast augmentation prefer a natural appearance. 'Protrusion' refers to how far forward the breasts project, as opposed to how big they are. Surgeon can order implants for their patients whose protrusions range from low to very high. The ideal breast implant size and shape for any particular person depends on their overall body shape and their own perception of personal beauty.

BREAST AUGMENTATION:
FAT TRANSFER

As an alternative to implants, the size of the breasts may be increased with fat transfer—also known as fat augmentation or fat grafting. 'Autologous fat transfer' refers to using the patient's own fat, as opposed to tissue from a human tissue bank.

The procedure involves removing the patient's fat tissue from another part of the body by liposuction and grafting it into the breasts. It is normal for fat to be present in the area of the breasts. Adding some extra fat can increase breast volume while looking and feeling natural.

Many patients ask their surgeons to remove the fat cells from problem areas such as the buttocks, stomach and thighs, which resolves two issues simultaneously.

The results of a fat transfer procedure may last for many years, or even for a lifetime. However, in some patients, part of the grafted fat may be reabsorbed by the body, thus decreasing the size of the breasts. It is not possible to determine, before the procedure, whether this will happen or to what degree. The probability of fat reabsorption can be decreased if the surgeon uses modern techniques.

To quote from the companion volume, '*Ultimate Beauty 1: Face and Skin*', 'Transferred fat survives when it gains a blood supply in its new location. This gives it a source of oxygen and nutrients, which permits it to continue existing indefinitely. If the transferred fat does not receive a blood supply in the first few weeks after surgery, the body will slowly break it down and absorb it. Thus the cosmetic improvements will disappear.

'Successful fat transfer surgery needs to be done with skill and precision, to make sure that the fat which is harvested is not damaged by the harvesting process, and that the fat is re-injected in a way that maximizes the potential for blood vessels to grow into it (neovascularization).

'It is to be expected that even when neovascularization occurs, it may not affect all the transferred fat, some of which will naturally be absorbed by the body. The amount that remains varies between individual patients, but generally about half of the injected fat remains for longer than three months. After that time has elapsed, the remaining volume of fat may last for years.

'If more volume enhancement is required then any harvested fat that has been stored can be used.

'Because the amount of fat retained by the body varies, some people need two or three treatment sessions to achieve the effect they want.

SURGICAL BODY RESHAPING
BREAST LIFT

A surgical breast lift is called a 'mastopexy'.

Many elements can contribute to sagging breasts. Aging, childbearing and weight fluctuations can cause the ligaments upholding youthful breasts to stretch and elongate, so that the breasts begin to droop. In medical terms, this is called 'breast ptosis', where ptosis means drooping or falling.

The goal of this type of surgery is to improve the shape of the breast by raising the nipple to a new position, removing loose breast tissue, and reshaping the breast to enhance its projection and its position on the chest.

Mastopexy differs from breast augmentation in that the purpose is to remove the excess loose skin. Often the surgeon will combine this with internal tissue shaping, using sutures, to help lift the breast from within. This may necessitate the removal of a small amount of breast tissue, but generally not enough to be noticeable.

To lift the breasts the surgeon cuts around the areola of the nipple and makes a vertical incision from the areola to the underside of the breast. Skin is cut away, creating a tightening 'lift' effect.

In a standard breast lift the surgeon does not actually remove the nipples. The incision that follows the circumference of the areola is only made so that the tissue surrounding the nipple can be reshaped.

If sufficient breast tissue is present, the surgeon may reshape it with internal stitches, remove excess skin and produce a higher, firmer breast. If there is not much existing breast tissue, an implant may be inserted during the lift procedure.

The surgeon closes the incision, generally using dissolving stitches to help minimize scarring. The procedure can take up to three hours. It is performed in hospital, with the patient under general anesthetic. The patient remains in hospital overnight.

SURGICAL BODY RESHAPING:
BUTTOCK SCULPTING

Surgical buttock enhancement involves either augmentation or recontouring of the gluteal region by one of three techniques:

- Liposuction (if the patient only wishes to reduce the size of their posterior). Learn more by visiting our section on liposuction, page 82.
- Liposuction and augmentation by micro fat grafting (if the patient wishes to reshape by reducing some areas and increasing others, without the use of implants). Drawbacks: the result of fat injection can be unpredictable in shape, and some of the fat may be reabsorbed by the body. Learn more by visiting our sections on liposuction, page 82 and body fat transfer (fat grafting), page 91.
- Buttock implants (if the patent wishes to increase buttock size and enhance shape).

BUTTOCK ('GLUTEAL') IMPLANTS

Implant surgery has become popular for men and women who consider that their buttocks are too flat, and who wish to have more muscular or shapely hindquarters.

The procedure can take place in a medical clinic, without the need for hospitalization. The patient lies on the operating table and receives a light general anesthetic. The surgeon makes an incision in each buttock and inserts the implant under the muscles.

There are major differences in how buttock augmentations are performed in countries around the world, and also in the types of implants available. These types include soft, cohesive gel implants, semisolid implants and the oval shaped implants designed by noted surgeon Dr. José de la Peña. Buttock implants can also be off-the-shelf implants or customized for a particular person.

BUTTOCK LIFT

Buttock lift surgery is designed to lift the buttocks without adding volume. The surgeon cuts away crescent-shaped sections of skin and fat from the top of the buttock and frequently from the sides as well. He or she then pulls the skin together and stitches it into place.

SURGICAL BODY RESHAPING: CALF AUGMENTATION

Men and women who are dissatisfied with the shape and size of their calves may seek calf implants. Calf augmentation is a surgical procedure that can:

- enhance the volume and shape of the calf muscles
- improve the proportions and shapeliness of thin or bowed lower legs
- correct asymmetry in calf muscles which may have been caused by an accident or genetic birth deformities.

The procedure is performed while the patient is lying flat on their stomach on an operating table and under anesthesia; either general, regional spinal or local.

The surgeon makes a small incision over the natural crease behind the knee. He or she introduces a long, blunt dissecting tool and uses it to create a pocket between the fascia (a layer of fibrous tissue) and the underlying muscle. He or she then inserts soft, solid silicone implants.

The incision is closed with dissolving sutures and after the surgeon has checked to make sure that the calves are both symmetrical, compression bandages are wrapped around the legs.

Calf implant surgery is a low-risk procedure; however as with any surgery there are potential risks and complications.

SURGICAL BODY RESHAPING: KNEE LIFT

Knee lifts are intended to reduce the baggy, wrinkly appearance of knees, which occurs due to the loss of elastic fibers, collagen, and muscle mass as we age. Knee lifts can be either surgical or non-surgical.

With surgical techniques, while the patient is under general anesthesia the surgeon cuts off excess sagging skin and may also remove fat, before closing the incision.

Liposuction is another surgical technique that can improve the appearance of baggy knees, especially if combined with skin excision. For non-surgical knee lift techniques, see "Non-Surgical Body Reshaping: knee lift" on page 104.

SURGICAL BODY RESHAPING: LOWER BODY LIFT

The lower body lift is also known as a 'belt lipectomy'.

During this procedure the surgeon removes excess, sagging skin. He or she then pulls up the remaining skin and stitches it in a new position to raise, tighten, and smooth out the surface of the abdomen, hips, buttocks, and outer thighs.

A lower body lift does not remove cellulite, but the fact that the skin becomes tighter and smoother means that cellulite's appearance is significantly reduced.

Disadvantages of lower body lift surgery include quite a lot of scarring, as well as the potential risks and complications entailed in any form of surgery.

SURGICAL BODY RESHAPING: THIGH LIFT

A thigh lift is a surgical procedure which involves removing skin and fat from the thighs to tighten the remaining skin and improve the contour of the legs.

This procedure generally takes two to three hours to perform. The patient is anesthetized, after which the surgeon makes the necessary incisions. These cuts may run all the way around the thigh, or only part of the way around the thigh in the groin crease, depending on how much of the thigh is to be lifted.

Next, the surgeon raises the skin and fat off of the underlying muscles. Excess skin and fat is cut away, before the remaining skin is re-draped across the muscles.

The incisions are closed using multiple layers of absorbable sutures which are positioned beneath the skin. A clean dressing is applied to the wounds and over this, a compression garment is worn. This compression garment helps support the legs during the healing process. It also aids in minimizing swelling and bruising.

SURGICAL BODY RESHAPING: TUMMY TUCK

A tummy tuck, medically known as an abdominoplasty, is used for patients who have loose or sagging skin on their abdomen after significant weight loss or pregnancy. While the patient is anesthetized, the surgeon cuts excess skin and fat away from the abdominal area and the sides of the abdomen. He or she also uses sutures to tighten the abdominal wall's muscles and fascia (a layer of fibrous connective tissue). After the area has healed, the abdomen will appear firmer and flatter.

SURGICAL BODY RESHAPING: LIPOSUCTION

Liposuction, also known as lipoplasty, liposculpture, suction lipectomy or simply lipo, is a cosmetic surgery operation that removes fat from many different sites on the human body. Patients may be placed under general, regional, or local anesthesia for liposuction procedures.

The physician must be careful not to remove too much fat. Excessive fat removal can cause the appearance of lumpiness or hollows and dips in the skin. Furthermore, the more fat that is removed, the higher the risk of adverse side effects.

It is not so much the amount of fat removed that can improve a person's appearance, as how well the body contouring has been performed. Skillfull liposuction may cause the appearance of weight loss to be greater than the actual amount of fat removed.

Areas of the body where liposuction may be performed:

- Abdomen
- Breasts
- Hips
- Outer thighs (saddlebags)
- Flanks (love handles)
- Buttocks
- Neck
- Back
- Inner thighs
- Inner knees
- Calves
- Upper arms
- Cheeks
- Submental area (chin, throat)
- Gynecomastia (male breast tissue)

PREPARATION FOR LIPOSUCTION

For two weeks before receiving any surgical procedure, the patient should not take any anticoagulants (anti-inflammatory medication). Patients should quit smoking for at least two months before surgery, because nicotine interferes with blood circulation and retards healing.

RECOVERY

Depending on the extent of the liposuction, patients need 'downtime' from work for between two days and two weeks. Patients will be given an easily-removed compression garment to wear for two to four weeks.

Pain can be controlled by a prescription or over-the-counter medication, and may last as long as two weeks, depending on the particular procedure. Bruising usually fades after a few days or up to two weeks later. Bruising is more common in people who smoke after surgery. Swelling will resolve in two weeks or up to two months, while numbness may last for several weeks.

RESULTS

Patients will observe noticeable improvements in body contours within days or weeks, as the swelling subsides. The final result will be fully realized between one to six months after surgery.

SIDE EFFECTS

As with all surgical procedures, there are risks and complications associated with liposuction, however, overall it is considered to be relatively safe and effective. A side effect, as opposed to a complication, is medically minor, although it can be uncomfortable, annoying, and even painful.

Temporary side effects may include bruising, swelling, scars, pain, numbness and limited mobility.

POSSIBLE COMPLICATIONS

'As with any surgery, there are certain risks, beyond the temporary and minor side effects. Your surgeon should mention them during a consultation. Their likelihood is somewhat increased when treated areas are very large or numerous and a large amount of fat is removed. The cosmetic surgeon should give the patient a written list of symptoms to watch for, along with instructions for post-operative self-care.'[46]

TECHNIQUES OF LIPOSUCTION

In general, during a liposuction procedure the surgeon removes fat via a cannula (a hollow tube, like a straw) by the use of an aspirator (a suction device). Liposuction techniques can be classified according to the amount of fluid injected to liquefy the fat, and by the cannula's mechanism.

* Suction-assisted liposuction (SAL)

Suction-assisted liposuction is the standard liposuction method. The surgeon inserts a cannula through a small incision in the patient's skin. The cannula is attached to a vacuum device. The surgeon carefully pushes and pulls the cannula back and forth through the fat layer, breaking up the fat cells, which the vacuum device then sucks out of the body.

* Ultrasound-assisted liposuction (UAL)

Ultrasound-assisted liposuction is also known as ultrasonic liposuction. During this procedure, a special-ized cannula transmits ultrasound vibrations through the patient's tissues. This vibration disrupts the walls of the fat cells, emulsifying the fat (i.e., liquefying it) so that it can be removed out more easily, by means of a suction cannula.

Ultrasonic liposuction is more effective than other liposuction methods at treating densely fibrous areas like the back, the abdomen after a 'tummy tuck', the breasts – both

46   Source: 'Liposuction,' Wikipedia. Article retrieved December 2014.

male and female – and body areas that have previously been liposuctioned. It takes longer than standard liposuction, but no longer than tumescent liposuction.

After ultrasonic liposuction, the surgeon uses suction-assisted liposuction to remove the liquified fat, or to transfer fat cells to other parts of the body, where they can plump up sagging skin and add volume.

Older ultrasound-assisted liposuction methods were associated with cases of tissue damage, usually from overdoses of ultrasound energy. Third-generation UAL devices avoid this issue by delivering pulsed energy and using a specialized probe that allows safer removal of liquefied fat.

Some doctors claim that this technique is better at removing fat than conventional liposuction. Ultrasonic liposuction is more selective; that is, it disrupts fat cells but not blood vessels, nerves or connective tissue. Because of this, patients recover more rapidly.

VASER® is a brand name for ultrasound-assisted liposuction. It stands for 'Vibration Amplification of Sound Energy at Resonance'. Vaser liposuction is also called VASERlipo.

* External ultrasound-assisted liposuction (XUAL or EUAL)

XUAL is a type of ultrasound-assisted liposuction in which the ultrasonic energy source is outside the body, transmitting the ultrasonic waves through the skin. This makes ultrasound-assisted liposuction's specialized cannula unnecessary. It was developed because surgeons discovered that in a few cases, ultrasound-assisted liposuction may cause minor complications.

XUAL can also potentially be more comfortable for the patient, both during the procedure and afterwards. It can decrease blood loss, permit better transmission of energy through thick scar tissue, and treat bigger areas. As yet, however, its effectiveness has not been conclusively proven.

* Power-assisted liposuction (PAL)

PAL employs a specialized cannula with powered movement, so that the surgeon does not need to make as many manual movements. These devices are easier for surgeons to control, permitting more precise and efficient fat removal. In other respects PAL is similar to standard suction-assisted liposuction.

* Twin-cannula (assisted) liposuction (TCAL or TCL)

Twin cannula (assisted) liposuction involves the use of a tube-within-a-tube specialized cannula pair, so that the inner cannula – the one that sucks out the fat – does not damage the patient's tissue with every forward stroke. The suction inner cannula moves back and forth inside the outer cannula to mimic a surgeon's manual stroke, rather than merely vibrating, as other power assisted devices do. This makes the task easier for the surgeon.

The presence of the outer cannula also helps the surgeon to be more precise when performing 'superficial' or 'subdermal' liposuction. An added advantage is that the cannulas do not get hot, meaning there is no risk of friction burns.

* Water-assisted liposuction (WAL)

With water-assisted liposuction the surgeon injects a thin, fan-shaped water jet, which breaks up the structure of the fat tissue so that loosened fat can be sucked out.

* Laser liposuction

Laser Liposuction is also known as laser-guided liposuction, laser lipo and laser-assisted lipolysis/liposuction. It is a
surgical procedure. This technique can benefit aging skin that
is low in collagen and elastin. Usually, when fat is removed
from beneath lax skin, the skin can sag and become baggy-
looking. Laser liposuction has the advantage of being able
to stimulate skin-tightening while removing fat. Addition-
ally, superficial skin problems such as cellulite or scarring
can also be improved by laser liposuction.

People who benefit from laser liposuction usually have
one or more of the following conditions:

- Excess fat in mild to moderate amounts
- Mild to moderate skin laxity

The idea behind laser liposuction is similar to that of
ultrasound-assisted liposuction. The laser is administered
through a fiber which is threaded through a microcannula
(very thin tube). Laser energy liquefies the fat in the target
area, making it easier to remove. It is then vacuumed out of
the body via a cannula. Some practitioners do not remove
the melted fat. Instead, they permit it to be absorbed and
eliminated by the body, over time.

Laser liposuction can treat areas of excess fat and improve
body contours. It is thought that laser liposuction can also
reduce bruising and bleeding, because it can also cauterize.

Laser liposuction trade names include SlimLipo®,
SmartLipo® and Smart Liposuction®.

There are two techniques of laser liposuction:

1. Fat breakup, collagen stimulation and fat removal.
This technique has 3 steps.

- a) The laser light is directed to the deep layer of fat in the hypodermis (the skin's deepest layer), to destroy the walls of the fat cells, permitting the fatty oils to escape, and breaking up the cells so that they can be vacuumed out later.
- b) The laser is then directed to the dermis layer, just beneath the epidermis. It heats the skin cells, stimulating them to produce more collagen and elastin. By this means the skin will become more elastic as the treated area heals.
- c) The third step is the vacuuming out of the cell fragments and oils.

2. Fat breakup and collagen stimulation only.
This technique employs only the first two steps described above. Instead of being removed by cannula, the cell fragments and oils are absorbed by the body.

This method is best for areas of very thin fat such as on the face and neck, or where the patient desires skin tightening alone.

* Tumescent liposuction
Older methods of liposuction surgery required blood transfusions because significant amounts of blood were sucked out with the liquefied fat. With tumescent liposuction (also known as 'tickle liposuction'), the surgeon injects local anesthesia into large volumes of subcutaneous fat.

This eliminates the need for general anesthesia or 'twilight' sedation. It also minimizes blood loss. Excessive bleeding is less likely to occur with tumescent liposuction, because the anesthetic fluid actually prevents bleeding. This makes the procedure relatively safe.

* SAFELipo

SAFELipo® is the trade name of a liposuction technique that includes both fat shifting and fat grafting. It is suitable for both large and small treatment areas. It involves three steps: fat separation, fat removal and fat equalization.

Fat separation

The surgeon uses specialized probes to separate fat globules from one another and from the surrounding tissue.

Fat removal

The fat cells, which are mostly intact, are sucked out. It is easier – and arguably safer – to remove the fat because it has already been freed from the surrounding tissues.

Fat equalization

The surgeon smooths and contours the remaining layer of fatty tissues. After liposuction fat removal, there are usually thicker and thinner areas of fat left behind, which creates an irregular look in the skin. Fat equalization is the performance of local fat grafts – that is, the surgeon removes the tops of the fatty lumps, reposition them in the dips and smooth them out. This step reduces the risk of complications such as skin irregularities and adhesions.

SURGICAL BODY RESHAPING: BODY FAT TRANSFER

'Fat transfer', also called 'fat grafting', 'autologous fat transfer' and 'fat injections', is a surgical procedure in which the surgeon removes fat from one part of the body and transfers it to another. It is minimally invasive, since only needles and cannulas enter the skin, through miniature incisions. The volume of fat transferred can vary from small – no more than a teaspoonful to be inserted in the tear troughs just below the eyes – to amounts large enough to plump up buttocks or breasts.

There are several advantages to using your own fat to increase volume in your body. These include:

- You cannot have an allergic reaction to fat tissue from your own body.
- The result feels and looks natural.
- Fat transfer, especially in large amounts, is cheaper than using synthetic fillers.
- Your fat can be stored frozen, if required, and saved for later re-injection.

Body fat transfer offers benefits to the following body areas:

Buttocks. The appearance of small or sagging buttocks can be improved. Sagging skin can receive extra support from insertion of your own body fat, which holds the skin out and up, giving buttocks a 'lift'. For the buttocks, the volumes of fat harvested and injected are much larger than in areas such as the face. Because of this, the surgery will take longer.

Backs of hands. When the skin on the backs of your hands is thin, your tendons may show through. Fat transfer can alleviate this problem.

Breasts. There has been concern that fat transplanted to the breasts may cover up breast cancers or make them more difficult to detect. This suggestion has not been proven right or wrong, but to avoid potential risk, your surgeon will not transfer fat to the breast itself. It is considered safe, however, to transfer fat to the tissues behind the breast. This may push the breast forward and give the effect of breast enlargement. Note that this small increase in volume is not the equivalent of inserting a saline or silicon breast implant.

Fat transfer: the procedure

The patient is placed under sedation and local anesthetic. The surgeon then injects a solution into the body area from which the fat is to be harvested. This solution makes the fat easier to extract. The surgeon then makes a tiny incision, inserts a cannula (thin tube) and vacuums out the fat. The harvested fat is put through a process called 'concentration' before being re-injected into the new areas of the body. The procedure usually takes about an hour and patients can go home afterwards. No special dressings or sutures are required.

Most people experience swelling in the fat-injected area, particularly the face, for a couple of days. The usual 'downtime' required (time off work) is 5 to 7 days. The doctor may prescribe a short course of antibiotics to reduce the chances of infection. If there is any pain it can usually be ameliorated with over-the-counter pain medication.

Fat transfer: the results

The body will naturally absorb some of the injected fat. The amount left behind varies between individuals but generally approximately half of the injected fat will stay for longer than three months. After that time has elapsed, the fat that remains is permanent.

Skilled and experienced surgeons will be able to inject the fat in such a way that it is more likely to survive instead of being absorbed. If the patient requires more volume, then any stored fat can be used.

Fat transfer: side effects

The scars from the fat extraction procedure usually heal very well and disappear after a few months. The tiny injection site wounds heal after about a week.

Any surgical or invasive procedure involves risks. It is recommended that before you go ahead, you should obtain a second medical opinion.

BODY RESHAPING:
MINIMALLY INVASIVE METHODS

Minimally invasive techniques of body shaping include lipodissolve and mesotherapy.

MINIMALLY-INVASIVE BODY
RESHAPING: LIPODISSOLVE

Lipodissolve is also called 'injection lipolysis' ('lipo' means fat and 'lysis' means dissolving). This term describes the technique of dissolving fat by means of injection.

Injection lipolysis is a nonsurgical body-contouring treatment which is an alternative to liposuction. The doctor injects drug mixtures, including phosphatidylcholine, into fatty deposits on the patient's body. These drugs break down the fat, which the body gradually removes. The skin tightens over the treated area as the fat is removed, so that there is no bagginess and looseness of skin after treatment. It takes time for the body to process the broken-down fat. For this reason, it may be up to two months before the full results are seen.

Unlike liposuction and surgery, lipodissolve does not require general anesthesia or sedation. Topical anesthetic (numbing) cream and anesthetic (laughing) gas may be used for the procedure. There may be soreness, swelling, bruising, and the temporary appearance of lumps after the treatment.

Lipodissolve is particularly valuable for the treatment of fatty pockets that do not respond to weight-loss diets and exercise alone.

The fat cells are permanently removed. If the patient later gains weight, the lipolysis-treated area treated will not expand as rapidly as it would have done without the treatment. The body tends to deposit the newly-acquired fat in areas that have not been treated.

Two to three sessions per area are required for optimal results. There should be a minimum of two months between sessions.

Trade names of injection lipolysis procedures include 'Lipostabil'®, 'Lipomelt'® and 'Flabjab'®

BODY AREAS THAT CAN BE TREATED WITH LIPODISSOLVE

The most common areas that are treated are the stomach, hips, back, thighs (inner and outer), sides of buttocks, lower buttocks, just above the knees, arms, chin, face, neck, cheeks and jowls. A limited area can be treated in a single session.

In healthy men, lipodissolve can be used to reduce chest fat. Female breasts cannot be treated because they are chiefly composed of glandular tissue.

Lipodissolve liquids can also be injected into lipomas (benign fatty lumps that can grow just below the skin) to dissolve them non-surgically. Lipodissolve can even help to decrease cellulite, in contrast to liposuction, which can actually worsen the appearance of cellulite by destroying the circulation to that area of the body.

Injection lipolysis has also been known to reduce the appearance of stretch marks by direct injection into the stretch mark itself, although the results from this cannot be guaranteed.

LIPODISSOLVE: HOW IT WORKS

Phosphatidylcholine (PTC) is a compound that occurs naturally in the human body. Its chief function is to help emulsify and break down fat and cholesterol.

During lipolysis, the physician uses very fine needles to inject PTC directly into the patient's unwanted fat deposits. It emulsifies the fat, releasing it in a soluble form. The body is then able to eliminate it via the normal processes of the liver and kidney.

The phosphatidylcholine that is used in lipolysis is derived from soybeans. It is chemically identical to the phosphatidylcholine in the human body; nonetheless, anyone who is allergic to soybeans should avoid lipolysis.

THE LIPODISSOLVE PROCEDURE

The patient lies down during the procedure. First, local anesthetic cream is applied to the treatment area and covered with plastic film. It is left for one to two hours, to absorb into the skin. Inhaled anesthetic gas (laughing gas) can also be used, because the procedure can be quite painful. The treatment area is disinfected before being injected with lipodissolve through a fine needle. Each area receives a number of injections, spaced about half an inch (1 .5 cm) apart.

After the procedure the patient is allowed some quiet, restful recovery time before leaving the clinic. Patients are usually given compression garments to wear, to help prevent swelling in the treated area and thereby reduce any after-treatment pain. It is recommended that patients have one to four treatments per area at two monthly intervals. After treatment with lipodissolve, it is important that patients drink plenty of fluids and massage the treated area every night for two weeks.

SUITABLE CANDIDATES

Lipodissolve is suitable for people who are seeking to reduce localized fat deposits (fat pockets or fat bulges) that stubbornly resist efforts at dieting and exercise. It is not used chiefly for weight reduction. It is a body sculpting technique.

SIDE EFFECTS

The most common side effects include temporary soreness, swelling, and bruising of the treatment area. This lasts around one week on average. Uncommon side effects include nausea, vomiting, diarrhea, fever, infection (rare), and prolonged bruising. There is rarely an allergic reaction to lipodissolve and no true anaphylactic reactions have ever been recorded. Any lumps that may appear are temporary and can be massaged out.

LIPODISSOLVE VS. LIPOSUCTION

Injection lipolysis and liposuction are different procedures. They both produce different results and involve different downtimes. The results from liposuction are much more significant than those achieved from injection lipolysis, and multiple areas can be treated in one session with liposuction.

The major advantages of lipodissolve over surgical liposuction include:

- No general anesthetic or hospital stay.
- An even, pleasing contour is achieved because final adjustments can be made towards the end of the procedure.
- Minimal bleeding and bruising.
- Shorter recovery time; rapid return to work and normal activities.
- No stitches are needed.
- As the body removes the broken-down fat the skin tightens over the treated area. The process is slow and the skin has time to tighten. Therefore, unlike liposuction, it leaves no loose, sagging skin.

LIPODISSOLVE VS. MESOTHERAPY

Mesotherapy and injection lipolysis are very distinct treatments. Mesotherapy is a procedure that involves injections of various vitamins, minerals, medicines and amino acids into the skin. Injection lipolysis also involves a series of injections, however, the key component of injection lipolysis is phosphatidylcholine which is used primarily for the dissolution of fat deposits.

Injection lipolysis is also deeper than mesotherapy as it is injected into the underlying layers of fat, and not the skin.

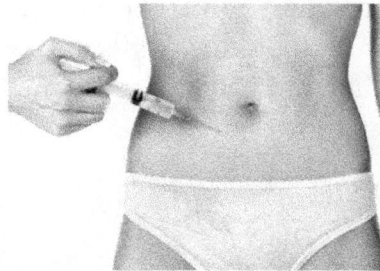

MINIMALLY-INVASIVE BODY RESHAPING: MESOTHERAPY

Mesotherapy is a minimally-invasive, non-surgical technique which was originally invented to relieve the discomfort and pain of inflammatory skin conditions such as eczema and psoriasis. It involves micro-injections of compounds such as fat-dissolving phosphatidylcholine, plant extracts, anesthetics, amino acids, vitamins, minerals, homeopathic remedies and enzymes into the mesoderm, or middle layer of skin. The ingredients of this 'cocktail' vary depending on the patient's individual requirements.

Mesotherapy advocates say that the technique can be used on the body to reduce pockets of unwanted fat on the hips, stomach and abdomen, outer and inner thighs, back, buttocks, knees, arms, waist and even hands. On the face, jawline, neck and décolletage it can be used to improve the appearance of wrinkles and lines, jowls and double chins, and fat pads beneath the eyes. It is also used for skin rejuvenation and may result in a slight improvement in the appearance of cellulite. See also "Minimally Invasive Cellulite Reduction: mesotherapy" on page 110.

A topical anesthetic cream may be applied before treatment, and ice may be applied afterwards.

After treatment, patients can resume their normal activities immediately.

Potential side effects may include a sensation of burning or itching, temporary soreness, some bruising. These problems usually resolve themselves within a few days. There may be a risk of swelling, infection, and irregular contours.

BODY RESHAPING:
NON-SURGICAL METHODS

Non-surgical techniques for body reshaping include microcurrent, acoustic wave therapy, radiofrequency, laser and fat freezing. Ultrasound may be used more commonly in the future. Body wraps can cause a loss of water from the body but they cannot remove fat.

NON-SURGICAL BODY RESHAPING:
LASER FAT DISRUPTION

Laser treatments can help remove fatty pockets and lumps from the body. Some trade names of laser fat removal treatments include 'Laser Lipolysis' and 'EndyMed® Fat & Cellulite Reduction'.

This type of fat reduction therapy uses light waves to target fat cells beneath the skin. Low levels of laser energy rupture the walls of the fat cell, causing the fat to leak out, without harming the surrounding skin, blood vessels and nerves around it. The released fat is then gradually processed by the body. Vigorous exercise after treatment speeds up the process.

NON-SURGICAL BODY RESHAPING:
MICROCURRENT COSMETIC
REJUVENATION

Microcurrent Cosmetic Rejuvenation (also known as electrotherapy) has been mentioned as a facial treatment in our companion book, *'Ultimate Beauty 1: Face and Skin'*.

Microcurrent is a non-surgical sculpting treatment for the skin, which can sculpt, lift and tighten the skin of the body as well as the face.

The microcurrent technique involves passing a very small direct electrical current (micro-ampere current) through muscle tissue. This stimulates healthy collagen remodeling inside the skin. Microcurrent cosmetic rejuvenation may also tone the muscle tissue by 'retraining' it.

After a microcurrent session patients usually experience no swelling, redness or soreness.

This treatment offers advantages for people who want quick results without the risk of surgery. There is little, if any, discomfort during the procedure.

It is recommended that patients attend a series of treatment sessions for best results. Patients may see some minor improvements after 3—4 treatments, and good results after 15—20 treatments.

Practitioners of this method say that if the entire series of treatments is completed and the patient attends regular maintenance sessions, the improvement should last 3-4 years.

Besides the face and neck, microcurrent cosmetic rejuvenation can also treat the stomach, legs, hands, back, arms, and buttocks.

Microcurrent is used for:
- Reducing the appearance of lumps and bumps on the body.
- Toning the muscles.
- Reshaping the body.
- Firming and tightening of loose skin and wrinkles.
- Lifting and firming the buttocks, stomach and legs.
- Reducing cellulite.

- Improving the appearance of rosacea, scars, acne, acne scarring and stretch marks.
- Improving the appearance of callouses on the knees and elbows.

Other skin resurfacing procedures stimulate collagen by injuring the deeper layers of the skin (dermis). Microcurrent does not work by injuring; nor does it require a period of healing to produce results.

NON-SURGICAL BODY RESHAPING: ACOUSTIC WAVE THERAPY

Acoustic wave therapy is a non-surgical method of reducing fat and cellulite. Acoustic waves are high intensity, oscillating sound/shock waves. These are emitted by a hand-held applicator. When they pass through the skin and penetrate down into the tissue of the lower layers, they can greatly improve the condition of weak and aging connective tissue. (See our section on collagen and elastin in the skin, page 63.)

Their action breaks down the connective tissue, releases clogged fat, stimulates nerves, greatly enhances blood circulation in the tissue and stimulates collagen production, thus strengthening and firming the dermis and epidermis.

Acoustic wave therapy was originally designed to disintegrate kidney stones without the need for surgery. Later research proved that the procedure could also help to alleviate the pain of soft tissue problems and calcifications (the accumulation of calcium salts in body tissue). Researchers discovered that it could also reduce cellulite and tighten the skin.

Acoustic wave therapy is suitable for patients with Grade 1, Grade 2 and early Grade 3 cellulite. Learn more about cellulite grades by reading the section on cellulite, page 36.

ACOUSTIC WAVE THERAPY:
THE PROCEDURE

The acoustic wave machine, when used to treat cellulite, has two different applicator attachments. Your esthetician will use the planar applicator (C-Actor) first. The head of this applicator delivers a high energy pressure wave with a very short duration of only nanoseconds. Because of this short duration, the high energy pressure wave is practically painless. The high energy has several effects:

* It breaks up the fibrous septae in the area that is being treated. 'Fibrous septae' are tissues that connect the dermis to the underlying layers of skin. The appearance of cellulite is caused not only by bulging fat pockets under the skin, but also by the fibrous septae, whose pulling creates 'dimple points' in the skin and giving the skin what is called a 'mattress look' or a 'cottage cheese look'.

* It stimulates collagen production in the lower dermis. The process also delivers some energy to the surrounding fat cells, disrupting their walls. This causes those cells to lose some of their fat.

After treating you with the planar applicator, your esthetician will stop the machine, remove the applicator, replace it with the radial pressure applicator (D-Actor) and resume treatment.

The radial head generates a pressure wave that is slower in duration, though still very strong. The slower pressure wave continues to break up the fibrous septae and boost collagen production. The radial head has actually been used in pain control. Its action increases blood flow to treated areas. When set to higher frequencies, the radial head can also increase muscle tone without you having to do any exercise!

Depending on the size and number of areas being treated, the procedure takes from half an hour to two hours. Patients need weekly sessions for 6 to 12 consecutive weeks. You should not have a break of more than a fortnight between treatments, because this can hamper improvement.

While undergoing the course of treatments, make sure you exercise regularly and drink plenty of water; this will help achieve good results.

After each treatment you might have slight discomfort, redness, or bruising in the treated area. This should resolve within a few hours. There is no need for any 'down time'.

People usually notice an improvement between the third and fourth treatment. Improvement continues for up to three months after the last treatment. It is recommended that you undertake a maintenance session once every three months thereafter.

NON-SURGICAL BODY RESHAPING: KNEE LIFT

Non-surgical treatments can never exactly mimic surgery, but they can produce noticeable improvement. Non-surgical knee lift techniques produce temporary skin tightening and smoothing.

A combination of infrared light, vacuum and bi-polar radiofrequency can be used to heat the deep fat cells of the knees and the surrounding connective and underlying collagen fibers. This causes a boost in circulation and cellular metabolism, with the outcome that the skin becomes tighter and firmer.

Generally, up to three treatment sessions may be required to achieve the desired result. The procedure takes around one to one and a half hours and entails little to no 'downtime'.

Trade names for non-surgical knee lifts include Vela Shape (TM).

NON-SURGICAL BODY RESHAPING: ULTRASOUND THERAPY

Ultrasound therapy is commonly used on the face and neck. It is not generally used to treat the body; however some doctors are experimenting with this.

The heat and vibrations delivered by ultrasound waves can warm up the layers of skin and deeper tissues. One effect is to increase blood flow, helping the skin to regenerate. Another effect of ultrasound waves is to selectively injure the skin, triggering a natural healing response. New collagen grows, and the elastin fibers straighten. In combination, these effects bring about a lifting, tightening and firming of the skin.

Ultrasound energy can also benefit the top layer of skin, exfoliating it, smoothing the texture and improving the evenness of skin color.

Trade names of ultrasound skin tightening systems include Ulthera®.

NON-SURGICAL BODY RESHAPING: FAT FREEZING

Fat freezing, technically known as 'cryolipolysis', is a non-surgical procedure designed to freeze the body's fat cells without damage to other tissues. The freezing induces 'lipolysis' – the breaking down of fat cells. Dead fat cells are then naturally eliminated from the body over the following months. There will be no noticeable difference straight after the procedure; it takes a few weeks for the treated areas to shrink. The treatment is safer than many other fat reduction procedures.

This procedure is best suited to people who are within 20—30 pounds of their ideal body weight, and who are maintaining or losing weight. The reason for this is that fat freezing does not actually remove fat from the body; it simply ruptures the walls of about 20% of the fat cells, which then release their fat from storage. The fat is gradually dispersed over several weeks. Your body treats this newly-released fat the same way it treats any fat that you eat; it uses it as energy or simply stores it again. So if you don't use up the released fat by exercising, or if you are gaining weight by eating extra food, the released fat will just be deposited elsewhere on your body.

This is not a weight loss procedure; rather, it is used to shrink stubborn fat pockets, for example bulges on the lower abdomen, the back or the hips.

The right candidate must not be too fat or too thin. They must have enough of a 'fat bulge' to grasp with the hand, but no more than a couple of inches (5 cm) thick. Fat freezing machines use suction to draw the fat between two cooling plates. If more than a couple of inches can be grasped, that may be too much to fit in the machine.

THE FAT FREEZING PROCEDURE

The machine holds the fat bulge in place by means of a strong vacuum. The cooling plates are set to the precise temperature at which fat cells will be permanently destroyed but your skin, nerves, blood vessels, etc. will not be damaged. The procedure takes one hour per treated area.

Afterwards, patients may experience some temporary numbness, moderate soreness and/or moderate bruising. No downtime is required. Generally, fat freezing is virtually painless, but rarely, some people may require analgesics.

After fat freezing, when the fat has been metabolized by the body and the bulge has disappeared, your skin will generally contract and tighten in that area. However, if your skin is particularly lax to the extent that it is thin and fragile, or displays severe stretch marks, or the abdominal skin droops like an apron, then it may not shrink back into place much or at all. Your health care professional will be able to help you choose a treatment for these issues.

FAT FREEZING VERSUS OTHER FAT REDUCTION TECHNIQUES

- Liposuction is usually more expensive than fat freezing, and involves some downtime. Sometimes the wearing of compression garments is required. The liposuction procedure, however, does remove fat from the body.
- Laser and radiofrequency cause the fat cells to leak, but do not permanently destroy them.

- Mesotherapy and lipodissolve injections are less effective than a single fat freezing procedure. They can be useful for people with unwanted fat bulges in areas of the body that the fat freezing machine's shape is unsuited for.

NON-SURGICAL BODY RESHAPING: ELECTRIC MUSCLE STIMULATORS

Electric muscle stimulating (EMS) devices deliver small, pulsed electric currents to the muscles. They are usually used as a form of therapy, to stop muscles from wasting away or to reduce painful spasms. Some of these devices are touted as 'bodybuilding' or 'muscle toning' machines which can make you lose weight.

EMS devices may be able to temporarily strengthen, tone or firm muscles, however the U.S. Food and Drug Administration does not endorse their use for anything except physical rehabilitation.

NON-SURGICAL BODY RESHAPING: RADIOFREQUENCY FAT DISRUPTION

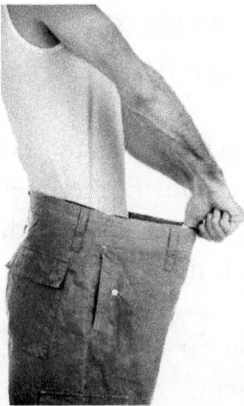

Radiofrequency fat disruption can help improve body shape and eliminate unwanted fat from areas such as face, neck, upper arms, abdomen, hips, knees, calves, ankles, male breasts, thighs and buttocks.

Radiofrequency delivers heat, via sound waves, deep beneath the skin into the fat cells, thereby rupturing them. Fat is released into the body, processed by the liver and eventually excreted naturally. A side benefit of this method is that it also serves to tighten the skin.

Radiofrequency should not be viewed as a weight loss procedure, but it is a good way to target fatty pockets, and thus contour the body.

Trade names of radiofrequency fat treatments include Vanquish® and Accent RF FatBlaster®.

See also "Non-Surgical Cellulite Reduction: radiofrequency (RF)" on page 114

BODY RESHAPING: CELLULITE REDUCTION

For introductory information, visit the 'cellulite' section on page 36.

SURGICAL CELLULITE REDUCTION: SUBCISION SURGERY

This is an older method of cellulite reduction that has also been used for years in the treatment of certain types of acne scars. It involves the surgeon making large incisions into the skin and using a surgical cutting tool to slice away the fibrous bands. The results, however, are not particularly good and the procedure leaves scarring.

Cellulite subcision surgery is performed while the patient is under anesthetic. The surgeon inserts a V-shaped tool beneath the patient's skin and moves it back and forth to slice through the bands of connective tissue which are drawing the skin downward and thus creating dimples.

Follow-up studies have indicated that this method gives long-lasting results. Disadvantages include the fact that it requires invasive surgery and does not work well for every patient or in every area of the body. Used in combination with fat grafting, cellulite subcision surgery is offered under the trade name Rejuveskin®.

MINIMALLY INVASIVE CELLULITE REDUCTION: MESOTHERAPY

Mesotherapy cellulite reduction involves injecting small amounts of medications, amino acids, and vitamins into the skin to break down the cellulite and improve blood circulation. Mesotherapy injections have been used to treat:

- acne
- aging complexions
- alopecia (hair loss)
- cellulite
- pain
- sagging skin of the face and neck
- scars
- stretch marks
- stubborn fat pockets
- wrinkles

Sometimes, mesotherapy is used in conjunction with wrinkle relaxants and/or dermal fillers to treat the appearance of facial wrinkles and lines.

Mesotherapy is considered relatively safe and most patients are able to resume daily activities immediately following treatment.

See also "Minimally-Invasive Body Reshaping: mesotherapy" on page 99

MINIMALLY INVASIVE CELLULITE REDUCTION: LASER

Laser Lipo Wand® Treatment is a minimally invasive procedure that, according to the manufacturer, results in "a dramatic and long lasting reduction in cellulite, that is clinically proven to improve cellulite by up to 80%" During the procedure the laser-liquefied fat and fat cells are actually sucked out of the body.

Cellulaze® is a trade name for a cellulite reduction procedure that takes around 90 minutes to perform. After the area to be treated is swabbed with disinfectant, the patient receives local anesthetic. The physician inserts a laser attached to the end of a cannula (a slim, metal tube) into the fatty areas below the skin, through tiny incisions.

The physician uses the laser energy to:

- dissolve the fat and remove any bulges.
- divide the fibrous bands so that the skin plumps out again.
- heat the skin and stimulate collagen formation.

No fat is sucked out, but the physician will apply gentle pressure to squeeze out any liquefied fat, which is then absorbed with swabs. Only one treatment is required, and the results are said to be permanent.

Depending on what grade of cellulite a patient has, (see the section on cellulite, page 36) patients can expect to achieve a reduction of two to three grades.

There is minimal downtime, with little scarring, and best results appear over six to 12 months.

MINIMALLY INVASIVE CELLULITE REDUCTION: LIPODISSOLVE

Lipodissolve or 'injection lipolysis' can also help to reduce cellulite. This technique should not be confused with liposuction, which can worsen the appearance of cellulite by destroying the circulation in the treated area.

Learn more by reading the section on 'lipodissolve', page 94.

NON-SURGICAL CELLULITE REDUCTION: ACOUSTIC WAVE THERAPY

Acoustic wave therapy, also called 'shockwave' therapy, is a non-invasive (non-surgical) method of reducing fat and cellulite. Acoustic waves are high intensity, oscillating sound waves that penetrate the deep layers of skin, breaking down connective fibers.

Trade names include SleekSKIN® Cellulite Treatment. This is a non-invasive technique that the manufacturer says "helps to smooth away the appearance of cellulite by stimulating the lymphatic system and strengthening collagen bands in the dermis."

During the procedure no fat cells are removed. For more information read the section on 'acoustic wave therapy', page 102.

NON-SURGICAL CELLULITE REDUCTION: ENDERMOLOGIE

An Endermologie® machine uses massaging rollers combined with vacuuming to reduce cellulite. The vacuum suction lifts the skin. This mobilizes the deep tissue, while the rollers simultaneously deliver deep, subdermal massage to the fibrous connective tissue and fat. This action releases the trapped fat.

The procedure can take 30 minutes to an hour, depending on the size of the area to be treated. For the best results, it is recommended that patients attend several sessions a week over a number of weeks.

NON-SURGICAL CELLULITE REDUCTION: HYPOXI

Hypoxi® is a system that combines gentle exercise with vacuuming. The manufacturers offer four different large vacuum chamber devices, each targeting a different area of the body.

The treatment takes place in one of several dedicated Hypoxi studios, where clients enter one of the chambers, or wear a special bodysuit, and proceed to exercise under the supervision of trained technicians.

Each session takes 30 minutes. This therapy is also used to target stubborn fat pockets.

NON-SURGICAL CELLULITE REDUCTION: RADIOFREQUENCY (RF)

Radiofrequency devices heat the area to be treated to a therapeutic temperature range, causing permanent destruction of fat cells in the target area and stimulating the production of new collagen.

This 'collagenesis' tightens your skin and connective tissue, whilst increasing your micro-circulation and assisting with lymphatic drainage.

The technique is non-invasive and requires no downtime. It can be used to treat areas such as face and neck, calves, upper arms, abdomen, hips, thighs, buttocks, knees, ankles and male breasts.

Radiofrequency treatments require a course of sessions, either weekly or fortnightly. Brand names of radiofrequency devices include Accent (TM). See also page 108.

NON-SURGICAL CELLULITE REDUCTION: ULTRASOUND

Low frequency ultrasound, delivered through the deep layers of the skin, causes the disruption of adipose cells (fat cavitation). In other words it breaks down the fat without affecting the surrounding vascular, nervous and muscular tissue.

The body then gets rid of the fat naturally. No anesthetic is required, nor is there a need for any downtime.

A series of treatments may be required. Brand names of ultrasound cellulite treatments include Ultrashape (TM) and Fat-Zap (TM). See also page 105.

NON-SURGICAL CELLULITE REDUCTION: COMBINATION TREATMENTS

'SmoothShape XV'®.

A combination of vacuum suction and mechanical massage with the emission of both light and laser energy can be used to treat cellulite.

The manufacturer says that the SmoothShape XV machine treats the underlying causes of cellulite through a proprietary technology called Photomology®.

'VelaShape'® and 'Velasmooth'®.

A combination of vacuum suction and mechanical massage with radio-frequency and infrared-light energy is used to stimulate collagen production and help reduce the fatty deposits that cause cellulite.

This procedure is similar to 'SmoothShape XV', but the added radiofrequency can also offer a skin-firming effect. The treatment feels like an intense, mildly warm massage.

Treatments every four to six weeks may improve the appearance of cellulite for six months.

VelaShape can be also used to tighten skin on the hips, inner thighs, stomach and abdomen.

Other combinations.

Cellulite can be successfully treated using a combination of ingredients which might include phosphatidylcholine (PTC, which is used in lipolysis), other mesotherapy ingredients and other non-surgical technology that not only destroys fat cells but also tightens loose and sagging skin.

CELLULITE TREATMENTS THAT DON'T WORK

Cellulite creams. It is claimed that these creams dissolve fat and smooth the skin. Many of these products contain aminophylline, a prescription drug used to treat asthma.

There is no evidence that these creams have any effect on cellulite. Their apparent effect may be due to the fact that they cause the blood vessels to constrict and push moisture out of the skin, which could be harmful for people with circulatory problems. Aminophylline can also cause an allergic reaction in some people.

Liposuction. This is a surgical procedure to remove fat deposits from the body. Liposuction, however, removes deep body fat, not cellulite, which lies just beneath the skin. The American Academy of Dermatology cautions that liposuction may actually increase the appearance of cellulite by creating more dimples and hollows in the skin.

Massage and spa treatments. Massage and other spa treatments may temporarily appear to make the skin look smoother, but they do not remove cellulite. Any effect is probably caused by the removal of excess fluid from the skin.

Body Wraps. These are said to work by extracting the toxins in the skin; however as for massage, any 'results' are probably due to skin dehydration.

BODY RESHAPING: SKIN TIGHTENING

Loose, sagging skin on the body can be tightened in a number of ways; surgical, minimally-invasive and non-surgical.

ⓘ SURGICAL SKIN TIGHTENING FOR THE BODY

Skin tightening for the body is best achieved by cosmetic surgery. It can be used to treat lax skin on the abdomen, back, arms and thighs. See the section on cosmetic surgery, page 68, for more information.

Skin tightening surgery for the body can include:
- Arm lift
- Back lift
- Breast lift
- Buttock lift
- Thigh lift
- Tummy tuck

② MINIMALLY INVASIVE SKIN TIGHTENING FOR THE BODY

There are several minimally invasive methods for tightening the skin of the face: there, however, may not be appropriate for the body.

They include:
- Anti-wrinkle injections such as Botox
- Dermal fillers
- Thread lifts

NON-SURGICAL SKIN TIGHTENING FOR THE BODY: LASER SKIN TIGHTENING

Laser skin tightening is a non-surgical procedure that requires no downtime. It uses a laser energy source to tighten skin by heating the collagen in the deep skin layers, causing the skin to tighten. Laser skin tightening is safe and effective for restoring a more firm, youthful appearance to skin all over the body. The result is noticeable straight after treatment. Further skin tightening takes place over the next few months as the healing process continues. For best results, two or three treatments about a month apart are recommended.

Laser skin tightening is appropriate for the reduction of fine lines, wrinkles, and skin laxity. The results cannot compare with the striking outcomes of a face lift, however, because laser is unable to address extreme skin laxity. The procedure, however, carries less risk of adverse outcomes than surgery.

Trade names of laser devices for skin tightening include:

- Polaris™
- Titan™
- Thermage™
- Lux Deep IR
- ReFirme™
- LuxIR™
- Aluma™
- Fraxel™
- LuxIR Infrared™
- EndyMed 3 Deep RF™

Each laser skin tightening system is designed to offer unique benefits. One system may be more appropriate for a particular patient's requirements than another.

Treatment times vary depending on the size of the area to be treated and the laser system used.

OTHER WAYS TO TIGHTEN BODY SKIN

Moisturizers and sunscreens help to preserve your skin's existing tightness and elasticity, so apply them daily. Weight training tones your muscles, which helps make the overlying skin appear tighter and smoother.

Body skin firming creams containing collagen or similar ingredients are unlikely to have any effect.

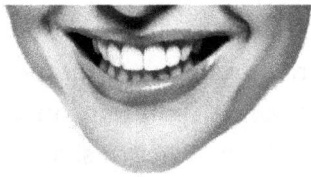

Part 5:
Teeth Therapy

TEETH THERAPY: TEETH WHITENING

Teeth may become discolored with extrinsic stains (superficial stains found on the surface of the tooth) or intrinsic stains (stains formed deep within the tooth). Tooth discoloration can happen for the following reasons:

- Food and drink, especially the consumption of tea, coffee, red wine and/or soft drinks over a prolonged period. These cause extrinsic stains.
- Smoking (extrinsic stains).
- Tooth injury (intrinsic stains).
- Age. No matter how well you clean your teeth, they will eventually become duller as you age. This is due to intrinsic staining.

METHODS OF TEETH WHITENING

* **Whitening toothpastes**: These are toothpastes containing active teeth whitening ingredients. They are best at removing extrinsic stains – those which are caused by the food and drink you consume, or by smoking. The important ingredients for whitening the teeth are baking soda and hydrogen peroxide. By regularly brushing with whitening toothpastes, you can prevent the gradual discoloration of your teeth.

* **Dental treatment:** Extrinsic stains on teeth surfaces can be removed by your dentist performing a professional 'scale and clean'.

* **Over-the-counter teeth bleaching and whitening formulas**: Teeth bleaching formulas are similar to teeth whitening toothpastes except that their active ingredients are more concentrated. They generally contain double or triple the amount of active ingredients. Teeth bleaching kits, which include a whitening paste and some form of applicator, can be purchased over-the-counter at drugstores/pharmacies, so that the treatment may be carried out at home.

* **Professional teeth bleaching and whitening formulas**: Teeth bleaching kits can also be provided by dental professionals, who can monitor the health of your teeth and gums before, during and after treatment. They generally comprise a mild bleaching gel in a custom-fitted tray that is worn over the teeth for several hours daily or nightly. Formulas used by dentists are generally more effective than the over-the-counter versions and may contain more hydrogen peroxide. For this reason, part of the kit usually includes some form of gum protection or gum shield.

* **Veneers**: These are porcelain facades that your dentist glues to your teeth. This facade covers up the existing, discolored tooth enamel. You and your dentist can choose your preferred color. This option is more expensive than the treatments mentioned above.

* **Laser teeth whitening**: These treatments are offered by cosmetic clinics as well as by dental professionals. They are advertised as a 'one-hour tooth whitening procedure with immediate results'. Teeth can be made six to eight shades whiter in a relatively short time. A whitening gel is applied

directly onto the tooth surface, after which a bright, cool light is shone onto the teeth. The light activates the gel, boosting the whitening process. Some brand names of this form of tooth whitening therapy include

- Brite Smile™ system.
- Zoom3™ Advanced Power whitening system.
- Beyond White Spa® system.

SHOULD YOU WHITEN YOUR TEETH?

Not everyone's teeth are suitable to be whitened. If your teeth and gums are not healthy before you whiten, the treatment can harm them. Even if there is nothing wrong with your teeth there may be other reasons why whitening is not appropriate. The best way to find out if your teeth are suitable for whitening is to ask your dentist.

NATURAL TEETH WHITENING

Practising correct oral hygiene is a good way to make your teeth look whiter naturally. Brushing and flossing your teeth every day helps remove extrinsic surface stains from your teeth.

A natural toothpaste can be made by mixing baking soda, glycerin and water into a paste, along with a few drops of antibacterial (e.g. sage) essential oils. For instructions on making home-made toothpaste, see our recipes section, page 181.

TEETH THERAPY: RESHAPING THE TEETH

Straight teeth can boost your confidence. The appearance of your teeth can be improved by professional dentists and orthodontists.

* **Veneers** are a dental procedure in which thin tooth-colored facings are glued to the front of one or more teeth. They can be a good option for patients with the following dental issues:

- Broken or chipped teeth
- Crooked, oddly shaped or misaligned teeth
- Crowded teeth
- Gaps between teeth
- Stained or discolored teeth

* **Dental implants** can replace missing teeth, which can benefit not only your appearance but also help you with chewing! Implants are dental devices that are securely anchored in the jaw, in the site of a missing tooth or teeth, where they biologically fuse with the jawbone. The dental professional then attaches a color-matched ceramic crown to the securely anchored implant. It looks and works like a living tooth.

It is even possible to replace all your teeth with implants.

* **Crowns** are custom-made dental coverings that fit over the top of your own natural tooth, covering the whole of the visible tooth in an artificial layer. They can not only improve the appearance of your teeth; they also provide stability for your teeth.

* Orthodontics.

- *Braces* can move crooked teeth into alignment. Modern methods involve the use of clear braces, which are less noticeable than the older metal ones.

- *Invisalign®.* As an alternative to braces, patients can have their teeth gradually straightened by using a series of clear, removable plastic trays, called 'aligners'. This avoids the necessity for metal and wires. Invisalign's manufacturers recommend that the aligners be changed every two weeks, and should be worn at least 20 hours per day.

- *'Inman Aligner'.* This is a removable appliance used to align front teeth. It employs a spring bar across the inner side of the front teeth and another spring bar across the outside of the teeth. These work together to move the teeth into a better alignment. It should be worn at least 16 to 20 hours a day,

* **Bridges.** Missing teeth, or teeth that are too badly decayed to save by capping them with a crown can be cosmetically treated with a bridge.

To make a dental bridge, the dentist first places crowns on the two teeth on either side of the gap where the missing tooth used to be. Then he or she fuses an artificial tooth into place between the two crowns.

The artificial tooth has no root, but it is anchored in place by the neighboring, crowned teeth, which are rooted in the jaw.

* Cosmetic dental contouring

Dental contouring is sometimes called 'tooth reshaping'. It is used to correct problems such as slightly overlapping or irregularly shaped teeth, small chips in the teeth, or teeth that are very pointy.

During the process, the dental physician files away small amounts of enamel (the outer layer of the tooth) on one or more teeth. He or she then alters the shape, length, or surface of the teeth, often 'bonding' (see below) a special tooth-colored material to the teeth to shape and sculpt them.

* **Bonding.** Cosmetic dental bonding attaches a tooth-colored composite resin to the teeth to reshape them.

It can be used to:

- Repair chipped or cracked teeth.
- Improve the appearance of discolored teeth.
- Close spaces between teeth.
- Change the shape of teeth.
- Protect exposed sections of the tooth's root caused by gum recession.

Cosmetic dental bonding is one of the easiest and least expensive of cosmetic dental treatments. Disadvantages of dental bonding are that the material does not resist staining as well as crowns or veneers do, nor does it last as long, nor is it as strong.

* **Dentures.** These days, dentures can be custom made to look very natural. With 'cosmetic dentures' the patient can choose the shade, shape, color, texture and position of their new teeth.

Partial dentures are also available.

TEETH THERAPY:
RESHAPING THE GUMS

Cosmetic gum reshaping can be used to improve the look of your smile, especially in the following cases.

* Gumminess

When some people smile, a large portion of their gums is revealed. This portion can vary from a few millimeters to an equal measure of gum and teeth showing. If people feel dissatisfied with this look, it can be treated with cosmetic dentistry. Your dentist or periodontist can reshape excess gum and bone tissue, to reveal more of the teeth and less of the gums.

* Uneven Gum Line

The best-looking gum lines have an even, upward curve from the centre to the sides. Some people have gum lines that are lumpy and bumpy. Again, the gum line can be cosmetically reshaped, if so desired. Your dentist or periodontist can create an even gum line across the front teeth, improving the appearance of your smile.

* Gum Recession or 'Long Teeth'

Sometimes, the teeth may appear 'long', even though they are, in reality, normal-sized. This look is a result of receding gums ('gingival recession'). When the gums shrink back, they expose more of the tooth's root. This can occur over time, often when people have been brushing their teeth the wrong way or using a toothbrush that is too hard, or when gum disease is present.

Your dentist or periodontist can treat this, either by grafting some gum tissue from another part of the mouth, such as the roof of the mouth, or by using materials from a tissue bank. Tissue banks store material that has been donated by other people and 'neutralized', ready for grafting.

Part 6:
Hair Therapy

In this section we look at baldness and thinning hair treatments, unwanted body and facial hair removal, and hair care and styling. Eyebrow grooming and eyelash enhancement are covered in the companion volume: *Ultimate Beauty 1: Face and Skin.*

HAIR THERAPY: PATTERN BALDING

Pattern baldness can affect up to 70% of men (male pattern balding,) and 40% of women (female pattern balding) at some point in their lifetime.

On men, this usually shows up as a distinctive pattern of hairline recession and loss of hair in a circle on top of the scalp, like a monk's tonsure.

Women normally display a general thinning of the hair over the top of their scalps or at the temples. For both men and women, losing their hair can be a frustrating experience.

CURRENT TREATMENTS
FOR PATTERN BALDING

- Excimer, helium-neon, and fractional erbium-glass laser therapy.
- Low level laser therapy.
- Therapy with oral or topical medications such as minoxidil (Regaine™, Kirkland minoxidil™ and Lipogaine™) and finasteride (Propecia™ and Proscar™).
- Camouflaging the problem with wigs, or by using special hair shampoos or ointments which coat the hair shafts and make the hair appear thicker overall, without actually causing more hair to grow.

- Using '*trompe-l'œil*' to trick the eye of the beholder, with scalp tattoos by skilled tattoo artists, which can imitate the look of a short 'buzz cut' hairstyle.
- Surgical hair transplantation.

* Laser therapy

Laser devices used to treat hair loss include the excimer, helium-neon and fractional erbium-glass laser.

One study has shown that laser light can stimulate hair growth at some wavelengths.[47]

However according to Choice Magazine[48], '… there's no definitive answer as to whether or not laser therapy works. It appears to stimulate follicles, and your hair will probably look healthier. However, clinical trials showing hair loss prevention and regrowth are [sparse], and the ideal laser wavelength, power, length of time and frequency of application hasn't been established.'

* Low level laser therapy

Low level laser therapy is also called red light therapy, cold laser, soft laser, biostimulation and photobiomodulation. It is a safe form of light therapy, used to treat pattern balding in both men and women.

Low level laser therapy (LLLT) uses devices with diodes that emit red light, available as:

- Bonnet or head caps.
- Hand-held devices.
- In-salon hoods or overhead panels.

---

47   *Lee, G. -Y.; Lee, S. -J.; Kim, W. -S. (2011). "The effect of a 1550   nm fractional erbium-glass laser in female pattern hair loss". Journal of the European Academy of Dermatology and Venereology 25 (12): 1450–1454. doi:10.1111/ j.1468-3083.2011.04183.x. PMID 21812832.*
48   *Treating hair loss: 1 Nov 2011. Author: Karina Bray*

Physicians hold varying views on whether or not low level laser therapy is effective at treating baldness.

* Medications

The first line medications used to treat male pattern baldness are minoxidil and finasteride. These drugs can be used simultaneously if necessary.

Minoxidil foam or cream, to be applied topically to the skin, is available over-the-counter without the need for a prescription. It should be applied to the scalp twice daily. It is believed that this drug helps strengthen existing hair, prevents further hair loss and (in some people) stimulate hair growth by increasing the blood supply to the hair follicles. It is most effective on people with recent or mild hair loss, but does not work well on people who have had significant baldness for a long time. It may be up to 12 months before you see a result, and if you stop using the medication its effects will immediately cease.

A number of other topical medications are also used to treat thinning hair and pattern baldness in both males and females, although this is not their 'official' use. They include:

- Dutasteride (trademark name Avodart)
- Ketoconazole, an anti-fungal which is also an ingredient in hair shampoos like Nizoral and Regenepure.
- Spironolactone and flutamide, both of which can be administered topically (by smearing onto the skin) or systemically (by taking the medication orally).

You get better results by using combinations of finasteride, minoxidil and ketoconazole than just using one of these drugs by itself.

* **Surgical Hair Transplantation**

With hair transplantation, hair follicles are surgically removed from one part of the body and grafted onto another. The 'recipient' area of the body can be the scalp, eyelashes, eyebrows, jaw (for beards), chest and pubic region. Rather than long strips of follicle-containing skin, numerous tiny 'plugs' of hair follicles are implanted in the scalp very close to each other. This results in a relatively natural appearance.

This is a popular treatment for male pattern baldness. It works because hair follicles that are genetically resistant to balding are transplanted to areas of bald scalp. After surgery, the patient should wear bandages for about two days.

Newer techniques of hair transplantation include the use of bioengineered hair follicles.

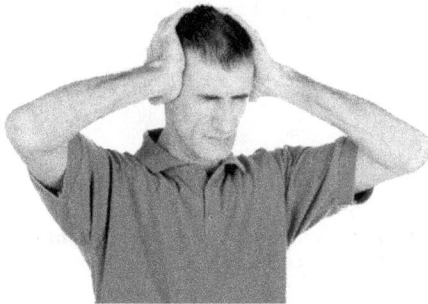

HAIR THERAPY: PATCHY BALDNESS

CURRENT TREATMENTS FOR PATCHY BALDNESS

A number of different treatments can induce hair regrowth in patchy baldness (alopecia areata), although they cannot cure it. Treatment is more effective in this type of baldness than in complete baldness (alopecia totalis/alopecia universalis). Your doctor will adjust your patchy baldness therapy according to your age and the severity of the condition.

First-choice therapies for patchy baldness include:

* Excimer laser

Treatment with an excimer laser twice a week for 12 weeks has been shown to produce hair regrowth in approximately 41.5% of treated areas, with no significant adverse side-effects[49]. Furthermore, the use of excimer laser in children with patchy baldness has a good success rate.[50]

* Fractional photothermolysis laser

Good hair regrowth may be achieved by treatment with a fractional Er: Glass laser.[51]

---

49   *Al-Mutairi N. 308-nm excimer laser for the treatment of alopecia areata. Dermatol Surg 2007;33:1483-7.*
50   *Management of alopecia areata: an update. Imran Majid and Abid Keen Cite this article as: BJMP 2012;5(3):a530*
51   *Yoo KH, Kim MN, Kim BJ, Kim CW. Treatment of alopecia areata with fractional photothermolysis laser. Int J Dermatol. 2010;49(7):845–847. [PubMed]*

* Intralesional corticosteroid injections

With this treatment, a doctor injects corticosteroid into the patient's skin at 4–6 weekly intervals. A number of studies have indicated that intralesional corticosteroid injections are efficacious. Abell and Munro noted hair regrowth in 71% of patients with alopecia areata treated by triamcinolone acetonide injections and in only 7% of a placebo group.[52]

* Topical corticosteroids

Many forms of topical corticosteroids have been prescribed for patchy baldness, including creams, gels, ointments, lotions and foams. Betamethasone valerate foam has been reported to be very useful. [53] Topical corticosteroids are much less effective in alopecia totalis and alopecia universalis.[54]

* Minoxidil

Doctors sometimes prescribe minoxidil 5% solution or foam, in conjunction with other therapeutic agents, to treat patchy baldness. This therapy does not seem to benefit patients with alopecia totalis or alopecia universalis.

---

52   Abell E, Munro DD. Intralesional treatment of alopecia areata with tri-amcinolone acetonide by jet injector. Br J Dermatol. 1973;88(1):55–59. [PubMed]

53   Mancuso G, Balducci A, Casadio C, et al. Efficacy of betamethasone valer-ate foam formulation in comparison with betamethasone dipropionate lotion in the treatment of mild-to-moderate alopecia areata: a multicenter, prospective, rand-omized, controlled, investigator-blinded trial. Int J Dermatol. 2003;42(7):572–575. [PubMed]

54   Tosti A, Piraccini BM, Pazzaglia M, Vincenzi C. Clobetasol propionate 0.05% under occlusion in the treatment of alopecia totalis/universalis. J Am Acad Dermatol. 2003;49(1):96–98. [PubMed]

Unwanted side-effects of topical minoxidil may include contact dermatitis.[55]

* Anthralin

Anthralin is a topical preparation which has to be applied daily at a concentration of 0.5%–1%. It causes a mildly irritant reaction in the skin, which in turn may cause hair re-growth. Its possible unwanted side-effects include serious skin irritation and staining of skin and clothes.

* Topical immunotherapy

Topical sensitizing solutions have been applied to the skin of some patients once a week, as a treatment for alopecia areata. This has moderate success. In one study when the treatment was stopped, patchy baldness recurred in around 60% of patients.[56]

* Prostaglandin analogs

Regular application of prostaglandin analog eye drops has been shown to induce eyelash regrowth in some people with alopecia universalis.[57][58]

---

55   Alopecia areata: a new treatment plan. Adel Alsantali. Clin Cosmet Investig Dermatol. 2011; 4: 107–115. Published online 2011 July 22. doi: 10.2147/CCID.S22767 PMCID: PMC3149478

56   Wiseman MC, Shapiro J, MacDonald N, Lui H. Predictive model for immunotherapy of alopecia areata with diphencyprone. Arch Dermatol. 2001;137(8):1063–1068. [PubMed]

57   Coronel-Perez IM, Rodriguez-Rey EM, Camacho-Martinez FM. Latanoprost in the treatment of eyelash alopecia in alopecia areata universalis. J Eur Acad Dermatol Venereol. 2010;24(4):481–485. [PubMed]

58   Vila OT, Camacho Martinez FM. Bimatoprost in the treatment of eyelash universalis alopecia areata. Int J Trichology. 2010;2(2):86–88. [PubMed]

* Topical retinoids (Vitamin A)

55% of patients treated with topical tretinoin experienced good hair regrowth. By comparison, 70% treated with topical steroids and 35% treated with dithranol experienced good hair regrowth.[59]

* Bexarotene

Some limited success has been reported in alopecia areata patients treated with bexarotene gel. Mild skin irritation is a common side effect.[60]

* Capsaicin

Capsaicin is a substance found in chili peppers. When applied to the skin (or eaten) it is an irritant, and elicits a sensation of burning. In one study, 9.5% of patients with alopecia areata experienced acceptable hair regrowth after 12 weeks of applying capsaicin ointment.[61]

Second-choice therapies for patchy baldness include:

* Sulfasalazine

Trial studies involving oral courses of sulfasalazine have had fairly good results. Sulfasalazine is an immune system suppressant and can have serious side-effects. The patient's health must be closely monitored during treatment.

---

59   Das S, Ghorami RC, Chatterjee T, Banerjee G. *Comparative assessment of topical steroids, topical tretenoin (0.05%) and dithranol paste in alopecia areata. Indian J Dermatol. 2010;55(2):148–149.*

60   Talpur R, Vu J, Bassett R, Stevens V, Duvic M. *Phase I/II randomized bilateral half-head comparison of topical bexarotene 1% gel for alopecia areata. J Am Acad Dermatol. 2009;61(4):592.e591–e599. [PubMed]*

61   Ehsani AH, Toosi S, Seirafi H, et al. *Capsaicin vs clobetasol for the treatment of localized alopecia areata. J Eur Acad Dermatol Venereol. 2009;23(12):1451–1453. [PubMed]*

* Photochemotherapy

Photochemotherapy is a technique in which the patient undergoes a treatment called PUVA-turban, two to three times per week.

PUVA-turban involves the doctor administering a topical, dilute psoralen solution selectively to the scalp for 20 minutes using a cotton towel as a turban. The patient's scalp is then exposed to ultraviolet A radiation.

PUVA-turban is effective in about 70% of treated patients treated for alopecia areata, although in some patients the disorder might recur later.[62]

Third-choice therapies for patchy baldness include:

* Systemic corticosteroids

Systemic corticosteroids (cortisone pills) are one of the commonly prescribed treatments for patients with extensive alopecia areata. Alopecia totalis and alopecia universalis do not respond as well to this therapy as patchy alopecia areata.

The use of cortisone pills is limited by their unwanted side effects, which can include high blood sugar, weight gain, high blood pressure, adrenal suppression, painful menstruation, suppression of the immune system, and skin disorders. Furthermore, the relapse rate is high – around 14% to 100%.[63]

---

62   Behrens-Williams SC, Leiter U, Schiener R, Weidmann M, Peter RU, Kerscher M. The PUVA-turban as a new option of applying a dilute psoralen solution selectively to the scalp of patients with alopecia areata. J Am Acad Dermatol. 2001;44(2):248–252. [PubMed]

63   Alopecia areata: a new treatment plan. Adel Alsantali. Clin Cosmet Investig Dermatol. 2011; 4: 107–115. Published online 2011 July 22. doi: 10.2147/CCID.S22767. PMCID: PMC3149478

* Cyclosporine

The success rate in improving alopecia areata with oral cyclosporine is 25%–76.6% but unfortunately this therapy can have serious side effects including nephrotoxicity (kidney damage), immune suppression, and high blood pressure. It also has a very high relapse rate – up to 100%. Furthermore it is thought that in some cases oral cyclosporine may actually cause alopecia areata.[64]

* Azathioprine

Azathioprine, an immunosuppressive drug, has been used to treat a vast array of autoimmune diseases. A pilot study of 20 alopecia areata patients treated with azathioprine showed some limited success.[65]

* Biologic agents: Tofacitinib citrate

Tofacitinib citrate is a prescription drug used to treat arthritis. Individual case studies into its effect on patchy baldness are promising but large studies have yet to be conducted into its efficacy.

PSYCHOLOGICAL SUPPORT

The causes of alopecia areata are considered to include psychosomatic factors. The loss of hair can increase the sufferer's emotional distress, which in turn can affect his or her self-esteem, body image, and self-confidence.

---

64   Ibid.
65   Farshi S, Mansouri P, Safar F, Khiabanloo SR. Could azathioprine be considered as a therapeutic alternative in the treatment of alopecia areata? a pilot study. Int J Dermatol. 2010;49(10):1188–1193. [PubMed]

It is important to offering psychological support alopecia areata sufferers, to boost their self-esteem and help them to adapt to the disease. Support can include:

- Educating the patient about the nature of disease
- Psychotherapy
- Hypnotherapy
- Antidepressant medications
- Support groups

UNWANTED BODY HAIR

Depilation means the removal of the visible part of the hair, which shows above the surface of the skin. The most common forms of depilation are shaving and the use of chemical depilatories. It is usually temporary: that is, the hair grows back

Epilation refers to the removal of the entire hair, including the part below the skin. Methods include waxing, plucking sugaring, epilation devices, lasers, threading, intense pulsed light or electrolysis. Epilation may be temporary or permanent.

As mentioned in the section on hair issues ("baldness" on page 51) there are different types of baldness. The treatment depends on the type.

HAIR THERAPY: PERMANENT HAIR REMOVAL— ALL HAIR COLORS

ELECTROLYSIS

With electrolysis, your clinician slides a miniature needle down into the hair follicle until it reaches the cells responsible for hair growth. A tiny current is delivered to the spot. This destroys the cells that cause the hair to grow. The treated hair will be released from the skin and slide out. Blond, gray and red hair removal can be achieved with this treatment.

Hair growth follows a cycle with three distinct and concurrent phases: growth (anagen), cessation (catagen), and rest (telogen). All three phases occur simultaneously; one strand of hair may be in the 'growing' phase, while another is in the 'rest' phase. After each hair completes the three stages it falls out and the cycle begins anew.

The hair's follicle is only susceptible to electrolysis treatment during the first and sometimes the second stage of growth. If a hair receives electrolysis during the last phase of growth it will have no effect because there simply is no follicle there to target.

There is no way of knowing which phase of growth the individual hairs are in. That is why electrolysis requires several regular, frequent treatments. If a hair misses out on treatment because it is in the 'rest' phase, and then is given enough time to re-grow, it will return again to the 'rest' stage where treatment is ineffective.

HAIR THERAPY: TEMPORARY HAIR REMOVAL— ALL HAIR COLORS

WAXING

Waxing is a process that removes the hair from the root. Generally, new hair does not grow back on the waxed skin for four to six weeks, although that depends on which part of the cycle your hair was in at the time of waxing (see "Hair's growth cycle" on page 51).

Almost any area of the body can be waxed, including eyebrows, face, pubic area (called bikini waxing), legs, arms, back, abdomen and feet.

Strip waxing (soft wax) is involves spreading warm wax thinly over the skin. A strip of cloth or paper is pressed firmly into the wax, thereby adhering the strip to the wax and the wax to the skin. The strip is then rapidly torn off against the direction of hair growth, as parallel as possible to the skin. This angle is important because if the hair follicles are disrupted by rough treatment, new hairs may become 'ingrown' and sprout beneath the skin. Ripping off the strip at too much of an angle can also cause bruising and other skin problems. As the strip pulls away from the skin, so does the hair.

Strip-less wax (as opposed to strip wax), is also called hard wax. After being warmed, wax is applied generously to the skin, where it cools and sets hard in a thick layer, encasing each hair. It can then be torn off without the need for cloth or paper strips.

This waxing method is useful to people with sensitive skin. Strip-less wax does not stick to the skin as thoroughly as strip wax does, and fine hairs, being sheathed in wax, are removed more easily.

The strip-less waxing technique may also be less painful.

SHAVING

Shaving is the trimming down of hair to the level of the skin's surface. It is usually done with a razor.

DEPILATORY CREAMS AND POWDERS

A chemical depilatory is a cosmetic preparation used to remove hair from the skin. These chemicals weaken the part of the hair that protrudes above the skin's surface, so that it can be scraped off. The formulation is generally applied to the skin, then after a waiting period it is scraped away along the with hair.

As the epidermis is also rich in keratin, the skin may become irritated and sensitive if the preparation is left on for too long.

Chemical depilatories are used primarily for the arms and legs. They should not be used on the face unless specifically listed for that purpose on the product's label.

Depilatory products are available in gel, cream, lotion, aerosol, roll-on, and powder forms. Common brands include Nair®, Magic Shave® and Veet®.

SPECIAL DEPILATORY GELS

Specially formulated gels may be massaged into the skin immediately following any epilation treatment that removes hair from the root. The gels target hairs that are actively in their growing (anagen) phase.

The area to be treated is usually waxed or plucked to begin with. Next, the area is cleaned up and any wax residues are removed.

The gels are then applied, one at a time. They are gently massaged in, and each one is allowed to remain on the skin for one minute.

Re-growth is usually reduced by approximately 20% following each treatment. Treatment should be repeated within three to four weeks for facial hair and five to six weeks for body hair. Eight to twelve sessions are usually recommended for blond, gray and red hair removal.

Brand names for Depilatory Gel Treatments include: Depilar®.

PLUCKING

'Plucking' or 'tweezing' refers to the process of removing hair by mechanically pulling the item from the owner's skin.

SUGARING

Sugaring, sugar waxing or Persian waxing is a method of hair removal that has been in use since 1900 BC. Tt is speculated that honey was the first sugaring agent.

Sugaring is often compared to standard waxing. During the process, a sugaring substrate sticks to and essentially removes hair without attaching to the skin. The substrate can be applied at room temperature or heated to a lukewarm temperature, minimizing the risk of burns. For this reason, sugaring is generally preferred over waxing when it comes to removing hair from larger areas of skin. Nevertheless, sugaring can result in skin irritation, sensitivity, and reaction. However, this can sometimes be prevented by taking an oral dose of anti-histamine. Sugar itself is otherwise hypoallergenic.

There are some distinct differences between home and professional-use sugar paste. The majority of commercial products contain wax, while home-made pastes often utilize sugar and other natural ingredients.

EPILATION DEVICES

An epilator is an electrical device used to remove hair by mechanically grasping multiple hairs simultaneously and pulling them out. The way in which epilators pull out hair is similar to waxing, although unlike waxing, they do not remove cells from the epithelium of the epidermis. Aside from the spring in early spring-type epilators, there are no parts in epilators that require regular replacement. Epilators come in corded, rechargeable and battery-operated designs.

Epilation can be painful to some people because, as with waxing, it involves pulling hair out of the roots. Because of the pain involved being particularly bad on the first epilation of an area, some people prefer to have the area professionally waxed first, then use epilation to remove regrowth.

THREADING

Threading is an ancient method of hair removal originating in the Middle East. In more recent times it has gained popularity in Western countries, especially with a cosmetic application (particularly for removing/shaping eyebrows).

In threading, a thin (cotton or polyester) thread is doubled, then twisted. It is then rolled over areas of unwanted hair, plucking the hair at the follicle level. Unlike tweezing, where single hairs are pulled out one at a time, threading can remove short lines of hair.

Advantages cited for eyebrow threading, as opposed to eyebrow waxing, are that it provides more precise control in shaping eyebrows and is gentler on the skin. It can be painful as several hairs are removed at once: however this can be minimized if it is done professionally.

There are a few different techniques for threading. These include the hand method, mouth method and neck. Each technique has advantages and disadvantages; however, the mouth holding method is the fastest and most precise.

PRESCRIPTION DRUGS

These drugs directly attack hair growth or inhibit the development of new hair cells. Hair growth will decrease until it finally stops. Hair growth will return to normal if the use of the product is discontinued.

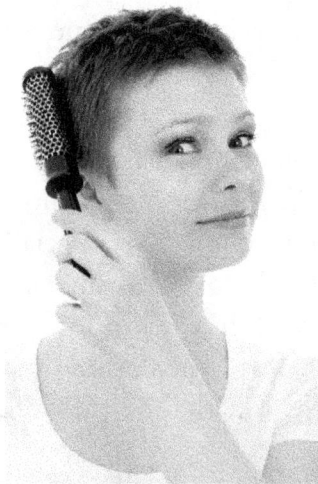

HAIR THERAPY:
BLOND, GRAY AND RED HAIR REMOVAL

Blond, gray, red and white hair can be removed from dark skin or pale skin. It can be removed temporarily or permanently.

PERMANENT BLOND, GRAY AND RED HAIR REMOVAL

The easiest hair for lasers to remove permanently is dark hair on pale skin. Laser energy is absorbed by pigment, so it works best when there is a strong contrast between skin and hair colors. It is not effective on blond, white or gray facial or body hair on pale skin or dark skin.

However, it is possible to permanently remove fair hair with other procedures, such as electrolysis, specialized epilatory gels or Intense Pulsed Light.

Intense Pulsed Light (IPL)

The wave lengths used by standard (older type) IPL machines target the melanin in the hair. Since gray, red, white and blond hair contains little to no melanin, IPL doesn't work. However, newer IPL machines have a separate head for pale hair that targets the hemoglobin (blood) at the root of each hair instead of the melanin.

First, the area to be treated is waxed. Waxing causes a microscopic injury to the skin inside the follicle, providing a target for the IPL and enabling blond, gray and red hair removal from pale or dark skin.

Some brand names of IPL for pale hair include Adena®.

HAIR THERAPY: DARK HAIR REMOVAL

Dark hair can be removed from dark skin or pale skin. It can be removed temporarily or permanently.

PERMANENT DARK HAIR REMOVAL

Permanent dark hair removal can be achieved by laser treatment or Intense Pulsed Light (IPL). Some brand names include Light Sheer Duet® diode laser, Starlux 500® (laser and IPL), Long pulse laser, Ulase® (laser and IPL), Q-Switch YAG Medlite® C6 laser, and Fotona® Dynamis laser.

DARK HAIR REMOVAL BY LASER

The easiest hair for lasers to remove is dark hair on pale skin. Laser energy is absorbed by pigment, so works best when there is a strong contrast between skin and hair colors. Choose a reputable cosmetic practitioner to ensure there will be no unwanted side effects such as burning or hyperpigmentation.

With laser hair removal, laser energy is used on the skin, focusing on the area of hair growth. The follicles beneath the skin surface are destroyed, stopping hair from growing.

A course of six to eight treatments is recommended to ensure the follicles are completely disabled and the hair will not regrow. Skin must be protected from sun damage afterwards or hyperpigmentation (darker patches of skin) may occur. After a course is completed, hair growth will be permanently reduced – and may stop altogether.

The advantage of this method is that any area of the face can receive effective long-term (and in some cases permanent) hair removal. The disadvantages are that the procedure is costly and takes some time. There needs to be a four-week gap between treatments.

DARK HAIR REMOVAL BY INTENSE PULSED LIGHT (IPL)

This is similar to laser treatment, but uses various light wavelengths (laser uses a single wavelength), which is said to reduce the risk of burning and pigmentation. Six to ten treatments are needed, with a hiatus of one to three months between each session.

After a course of treatments, hair may be expected to permanently disappear, or to be sparser and re-grow looking less coarse. As well as the permanency of the procedure, it is said to be a gentler, more comfortable form of light therapy.

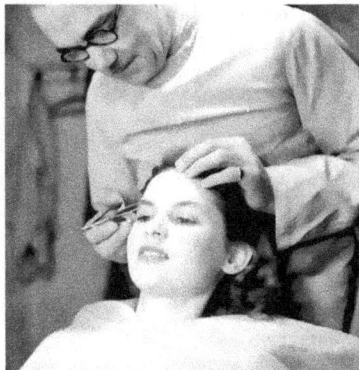

HAIR THERAPY:
HAIR CARE AND STYLING

It has been said that a person's overall personal appearance has three main elements; the body, the face and the hair on their head; and that the secret to looking good is for at least two out of three of these elements to be in great shape.

Bodies and faces are largely determined by genes and age, though nutrition and lifestyle play an important role. The easiest and quickest of these three components to control is your hair. Proper hair care and styling can make your locks look beautiful.

The appearance of the hair on your head has several components of its own:

- Texture—are the hairs fine or coarse, smooth or rough, curly or straight?
- Color—natural hair colors range from jet black through brown and auburn to blond, gray and white. Hair dyes have an almost limitless range of colors.
- Shape—by this we mean the overall shape of your hairstyle. It may be upstanding, wide, long, short, shaved, voluminous etc.
- Style—For example page-boy, mullet beehive, bouffant, tousled, quiffed, crimped, permed,
- Balance: oily, normal or dry
- Condition: healthy or damaged by sun, ill-health, chemicals etc.
- Abundance—plentiful, thick hair or sparse hair.

HAIR GROWTH RATE

Hair grows faster in warmer weather.[66] Hair growth rate also fluctuates with changes in our hormone levels. Numerous solutions have been proffered to increase the rate at which hair grows, including the application of herbs, eggs, 'nourishing oils' etc. Of these, two are most likely to be successful:

- scalp massage
- a nutritious diet

Scalp massage

Massage increases blood flow to the scalp. This technique involves using the fingers and hands to rub, knead and apply pressure to the skin of the scalp. Increased blood flow may nourish the growing roots of the hair follicles, no matter which 'nourishing oils' are applied.

Nutritious Diet

The cells that make up each strand of hair require a regular supply of key nutrients. An overall balanced diet is necessary for a healthy scalp and healthy hair. A lack of zinc, for example, can lead to hair loss and a dry, flaky scalp.

For healthy hair your food should contain protein iron vitamins C, E and A, omega 3 fatty acids, zinc, selenium and biotin. All of these nutrients can be supplied by fresh fruit and vegetables, legumes, whole grains, nuts and seeds.

---

66   'Seasonal changes in human hair growth' VALERIE A. RANDALL and F. J. G. EBLING Article first published online: 29 JUL 2006 DOI: 10.1111/j.1365-2133.1991.tb00423.x

HAIR HEALTH

The living part of the hair, the root or follicle is the part that is affected by massage and diet. It is also the invisible part. The strands of hair that are visible, the hair shafts, are actually no longer alive. Diet and massage will not affect them. Other treatments will, however. This is where those 'nourishing oils' come into play. Hair shafts that are in good condition would look smooth under a microscope.

Shine

Hair shine depends on the condition of the hair cuticle. The cuticle is the hair shaft's outermost layer. It is formed from dead cells which overlap, like scales. The cuticle of shiny, healthy hair-shafts is smooth and intact, with closely overlapping scales. It is the smoothness of the overlapping scales that reflects light, making hair look shiny.

Everyday grooming activities such as combing and brushing, slough off some of these cuticular scales. The older section at the end of the hair shaft usually has more scales missing. The process of losing scales is called 'weathering'. It is made worse by vigorous brushing and combing, and by the application of chemicals. Dyed or permanently waved hair has to have a disrupted cuticle in order for the waving lotion or dye to penetrate. The greater the damage to the cuticle, the duller the hair looks.

Softness

Healthy hair feels smooth and soft. Hair that has been damaged feels rough and harsh. Again, this is due to the condition of the cuticle. Hair shafts with an undamaged cuticle have a smooth surface.

Frizziness

Frizzy hair is a sign of cuticular damage. The shafts of frizzy hair tend to accumulate static electricity, because they gain a tiny electrical charge if the cuticle is broken. This causes the hairs to fly apart and separate, especially at the ends.

KEEPING HAIR HEALTHY

Hair breakage is one of the most common forms of hair loss. It commonly results from chemical processing or overly vigorous brushing or combing. Anything you do to your hair can cause damage to the shafts. Nonetheless, you can reduce injury by being careful with grooming, shampooing, conditioning, styling, perming and coloring methods.

Grooming

Never brush or comb your hair when it is wet. Wet hair is more easily damaged than dry hair. While it is still damp, untangle it with your fingers, then allow it to dry slightly before using a wide-toothed comb. Brushes are not suitable for untangling hair because they are likely to tear and break the hair shaft. As a rule, keep all grooming to a minimum. The less you mess with your hair, the less chance there is for damage.

Combs are better than brushes because they have less surface area to create friction and break hair shafts.

Choose a comb with smooth, widely spaced teeth. If you do use a brush, choose one whose bristles are widely spaced and have rounded tips. Any brush or comb that feels rough when you stroke it across the palm of the hand is probably going to damage your hair.

Shampooing

Sebum is an oily substance secreted by the glands in our bodies. It helps prevent hair and skin from drying out. Small amounts of sebum on the hair shaft are excellent for smoothing the scales on the cuticle and reducing static electricity.

The right amount of sebum makes the hair look shiny, decreases frizz and makes hair lie smoothly against the scalp.

The downside of sebum for people with fine or thinning hair is that it makes the hair look less full; instead it loses volume and looks lank.

The action of shampooing causes friction between hair shafts, which leads to avoidable hair fracture. Hair should be shampooed only when it is necessary to wash away dirt or excess sebum. You do not need to shampoo every day, especially if you have normal sebum production and your lifestyle doesn't involve spending time in a polluted environment.

For best outcomes choose hair shampoos that are non-allergenic, fragrance free and not tested on animals. See the recipes section, page 181, for directions on making your own hair shampoo at home.

Conditioning

Using conditioners after shampooing can be useful to people with damaged hair. Conditioner can minimize hair loss by untangling the hair and decreasing friction between the comb and the hair shafts as well as between individual hair shafts. Conditioner works the same way as sebum—by protectively covering the hair shaft. Unlike sebum, however, conditioners are designed to avoid giving the hair a greasy look or lack of volume.

For a simple, natural, highly effective conditioner that has emollient, humectant and emulsifier, use a few drops of vegetable glycerin, massaged into damp hair, especially at the ends.

Vegetable glycerin is so safe and gentle that it actually can be eaten, and is often used as a food ingredient. Do not apply too much, or your hair may become over-conditioned and look lank. Other simple, natural leave-in conditioning compounds include argan oil (aka Moroccan oil).

Many commercial conditioners include a synthetic ingredient called dimethicone. Dimethicone is a type of silicon oil. Instead of penetrating the hair shafts and nourishing them deeply, like natural detanglers, it coats the hair shafts, forming a chemical barrier.

For best outcomes choose hair conditioners that are non-allergenic, fragrance free and not tested on animals.

Drying

It is essential to dry your hair carefully to avoid breakage. Do not rub the hair vigorously with a towel. Rubbing the hair shafts together while they are wet generates a great deal of friction, which causes the shafts to break. Instead, blot your hair dry or wrap it in a towel to absorb some of the moisture.

Don't blow dry hair too frequently. Frequent blow drying, or use of other heat products, can stress your hair. If possible, allow your hair to dry without applying heat. The heat from blow dryers damages hair, causing frizziness. When hair is damaged it becomes weaker, and more prone to breakage.

If you really must use a blow dryer, switch it to the lowest heat setting and hold the nozzle at least 6 inches (15 cm) from your scalp. It is possible to buy 'vented' blow-drying brushes, which are designed to avoid high temperatures caused by heat buildup.

Do not sleep with wet hair. It is more prone to bacterial or fungal infection. It will cause an unnecessary increase of blood flow in the scalp as your body's way of protecting itself from bacteria. A reaction occurs on the scalp which can lead to a headache.

Do not comb, brush or style your hair until it has ceased to be dripping wet and is only damp.

Styling

The most effective way to avoid hair damage is to keep styling to a minimum. To reduce risk of breakage, hairstyles should be loose and not fixed into place with numerous hairpins or combs. Hair styles that pull at the hair, such as tight ponytails or cornrows, may break weak hair shafts.

- Choose barrettes that are rubber coated and have smooth edges. This will reduce hair breakage when the clasp is closed. Do not tie up your hair with rubber bands.
- Rubber bands should not be used because they are difficult to remove and cause unnecessary damage.
- Choose styling products that are non-allergenic, fragrance free and not tested on animals.

Coloring

All hair dyes weaken hair shafts, although some coloring techniques cause less harm than others.

Usually, darkening your hair is less harmful than lightening it. The first step in lightening involves a bleaching procedure to open up the cuticular scales. The second step is the dyeing. The bleaching and dyeing combined is more damaging than merely dyeing the hair. If you keep your hair color close to your natural color, you will have less damage. The more dramatic the color change, the greater the hair damage.

For best outcomes choose coloring products that are non-allergenic, fragrance free and not tested on animals. Hair can be lightened with chamomile tea or lemon juice. Red tints can be imparted with henna. Rosemary, sage and nettle can darken brown hair by a few shades, while black walnut powder can make it really dark.

Permanent Waving ('perming')

Permanent waving causes more damaging than dyeing because the treatment actually breaks down the protein structure of the hair shaft, then rebuilds it in a new shape. If you have your hair 'permed', remember that the shorter the treatment process, the less damage is caused.

If you intend to both perm and dye your hair, wait at least ten days between the procedures to allow your hair to recover somewhat. Also, make sure you do the permanent waving first, before the dyeing. If you color your hair before perming, you will cause excessive hair cuticle damage and significantly weaken your hair shafts.

Cutting and trimming

Trimming off split ends makes your hair look healthier because you have removed the older and drier end-sections of the hair shaft. Contrary to rumor, trimming does not make hair grow faster.

Part 7:
Fingernails and Toenails

Problems with fingernails and toenails can be indicators of underlying illnesses or nutritional deficiencies, so see your doctor straight away if your nails —

- are loose and separated from the nail bed (onycholysis).
- have indentations running across them (Beau's lines).
- have a dark band across the top (Terry's nails).
- are soft and looked like scooped-out spoons (koilonychia).
- curve around your fingertips, which are becoming enlarged (club nails).
- are pitted with small dents.
- are thick and slow-growing, and look yellowish (yellow nail syndrome).
- are extremely pale and whitish.
- have dark brown or black vertical lines (possible melanoma).
- are bluish in color for a prolonged period.
- have unexplained bleeding, redness, swelling or pain.

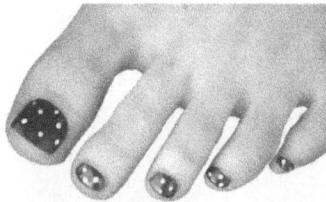

ABOUT FINGERNAILS AND TOENAILS

Our fingernails and toenails, which are made of a protein called keratin, grow at a rate of approximately 0.004 inches (0.1 millimeters) per day. If a nail is lost, through injury or disease, it can be up to six months before it grows back completely.

Each nail has six parts.

- The *nail fold* is the ridge of skin that surrounds each nail.
- The *nail plate* is the visible part; that which we usually call a fingernail or toenail.
- The *nail bed* lies beneath the nail plate. Its job is to nourish the nail.
- The *lunula* is the paler, crescent-shaped area at the base of the nail. It is part of the nail matrix.
- The *cuticle* is the tissue overlapping the nail at its base.
- The *nail matrix* is hidden underneath the cuticle. Situated at the base of the nail, it is a fold of skin composed largely of dead cells. Its job is to prevent the entry of bacteria and to manufacture new nail cells.

FINGERNAILS AND TOENAILS: HOW TO KEEP THEM HEALTHY

BE HYGIENIC

Keep your nails clean and dry. Bacteria, fungi and other nasties thrive in damp, dirty conditions, and they can actually grow under your fingernails if the conditions are right for them.

BE GENTLE ON YOUR NAILS

Nails are only small pieces of keratin protecting the tips of your fingers and toes. If you use your nails as tools, for example to pry open containers or pick at hard objects, you risk damaging them.

Do not nibble or bite your fingernails, or scrape at your cuticles. These activities may injure the nail bed. Bacteria and fungi can easily enter broken skin; even a small cut can cause infection.

If you have a hangnail (see 'hangnails', below) cut it off with sharp scissors. Do not try to pull it off, as you may tear the skin.

GO POLISH-FREE—OR USE POLISH THAT IS CERTIFIED BY THE CAMPAIGN FOR SAFE COSMETICS

Nail polish (also called nail varnish or nail lacquer) can harm not only your health but also the health of the environment. It is far from being a natural product and is manufactured from a number of potent chemicals.

Until around 2007, most commercial nail polish formulas contained a range of toxic substances such as formaldehyde, toluene and dibutyl phthalate (DBP).

- Formaldehyde can cause cancer in humans. It can also irritate the eyes, throat, nose and skin.
- DBP is used in nail polishes as a dye solvent for dyes and to prevent the product from becoming brittle.

It is easily absorbed through the skin and has been shown to be toxic to the reproductive organs, to reduce sperm count and to harm the development of unborn children. In 2005 the European Union banned the use of DBP in personal products, though other countries continued to tolerate it.

- Toluene, too, may damage reproductive systems and interfere with the development of children. It can also lead to headaches, dizziness and fatigue.

All these chemicals are readily absorbed into the body through the porous material of the nails and the nail bed.

Due to activism from the Campaign for Safe Cosmetics, after 2007 a number of leading international companies stopped adding those three chemicals to their nail polish.

Nonetheless, there are still plenty of manufacturers who continue to use them. Check the label on your nail polish bottle.

Even nail polishes that do not contain those three poisons may contain other potentially dangerous chemicals, such as chemical dyes, ethyl acetate, or isopropyl alcohol.

Some people may also have allergic reactions to some of the less toxic chemicals in nail polishes and polish removers.

When old bottles of nail polish are thrown into the trash, the toxic compounds they contain end up in landfill. From there they percolate into the soil and groundwater, poisoning the environment.

If you care about your health and the environment but still want colorful, glittery or super-shiny nails, seek products made by companies who have signed up with the Campaign for Safe Cosmetics. As a further precaution, do not wear nail polish all the time. Take a holiday from it occasionally. When you remove it, choose acetone-free nail polish remover.

Alternatively, go polish-free. Healthy, clean nails are beautiful and, in the opinion of many, need no other adornment. Another great reason to go polish-free is that you won't have to use nail polish remover, with all its potentially harmful chemicals.

If you are keen on decorating your nails the no-polish way, try using stick-on nail decorations, also called nail transfers or nail wraps. These stickers are generally made of plastic or foil, and are available in a variety of designs. They can be bought from cosmetics stores (check the labels to make sure there are no toxic chemicals in the glue) and they even come in 'transparent', to give nails that extra shine.

Some people buff their nails as a no-polish alternative to making their nails look shiny. This carries its own disadvantages—see the section entitled 'Avoid Buffing your Nails', page 168.

BEWARE OF NAIL POLISH REMOVER

Acetone is a chemical that was the chief ingredient of nail polish remover for many years. It not only strips off nail polish—it also strips away the natural coating of the nails, making them prone to brittleness.

Avoid acetone. Nail polish removers contain other chemicals, too, which can seep into the skin surrounding the nails.

PROTECT YOUR HANDS AND NAILS

Wear gloves when you are undertaking tasks in which your hands may come into contact with chemicals or dirt—for example when you are gardening, washing the dishes or cleaning your house.

MOISTURIZE HANDS, NAILS AND CUTICLES

Your cuticles act like a rubber sealing-ring, keeping out harmful germs from your nails. If you damage them, for example by picking at them cutting them or pushing them back too far, you will create an entry-point for infection.

Don't mess with your cuticles; nature knows best! To keep them in good condition, apply moisturizer regularly. Choose products that contain humectants such as urea, phospholipids and lactic acid. Humectants attract moisture. They help keep your cuticles and nails from drying out and cracking. (Lotions containing humectants are good for your hands, too.)

AVOID NAIL-HARDENING PRODUCTS

Many products that are sold as 'nail hardeners' may actually damage the nails. Avoid using them unless your nails are extremely soft and delicate. Very soft nails may be a sign of underlying diseases, so check with your doctor. Also, to avoid making your nails any softer, protect them from hot water and harsh chemicals.

USE FINE-GRAINED NAIL FILES

Do not use rough, sandpapery emery boards to file your nails. They can crack edges of the nail plate, leading to tears and breakages. Opt for delicate, fine-grained files instead.

FILE NAILS TOWARDS THE MIDDLE

When you file your nails, do not use a back-and-forth sawing action. File in one direction – away from the edge of the nail and towards the middle. When one side is done, file the other side of the nail the same way. Use slow, even sweeps of the file and be gentle on your nails.

KEEP NAILS TRIMMED

The fashion for elongated claws comes and goes. One problem with having very long nails is that is makes ordinary tasks—such as typing, or picking up small objects—more difficult to perform.

Trimming your nails regularly helps you to avoid snagging or breaking them. People whose nails grow rapidly will need to trim them more often.

Use sharp manicure scissors or clippers to cut your nails straight across, then clip the corners to 'round' the tips in a gradual curve. Smooth the clipped edges with a fine file.

Do not trim your nails to a pointed shape, and do not leave sharp corners on them—they will be more likely to become snagged on fabric or other things, and tear.

Leave a little bit of white at the tips of your nails. Cutting too close to the nail bed can allow the entry of infection, as well as making it difficult to pick up certain objects such as coins.

Some people prefer to trim their toenails when they are soft, for example after bathing.

LOOK AFTER YOUR TOENAILS AS WELL AS YOUR FINGERNAILS

The same principles apply to your toenails as to your fingernails. In fact, it is even more important to keep your toenails clean and dry because in the moist, dark enclosure of your shoes, fungus is more likely to take hold.

CHOOSE A GOOD PEDICURIST

If you regularly visit a professional pedicurist, ensure that the tools they use have been properly sterilized. A good pedicurist or trained podiatrist will never dig beneath the nail with sharp instruments, or damage the cuticle. They should cut the toenails straight across, and never at an angle.

AVOID HARSH CHEMICALS AND HOT WATER

Chemicals such as household cleaners and dish-washing detergents can have a weakening effect on nails, particularly if you use them often. Immersion in hot water can also have a drying effect on the skin and nails. Wear cotton-lined protective gloves when performing tasks that involve chemicals and hot water.

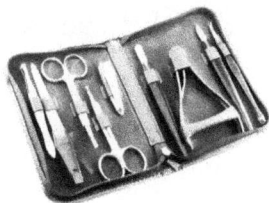

USE A NAIL BRUSH TO CLEAN YOUR NAILS

Do not use long, sharp metal tools to clean out the dirt from beneath your nails. This can produce a pocket between the nail plate and the nail bed, which is open to infection. Instead, scrub your nails gently with a nail brush.

AVOID BUFFING YOUR NAILS

Nail buffing is the act of polishing the nail-plate in order to make the surface look smooth and shiny. This practice is not recommended, because every time you buff your nails you are wearing away the nail surface, and making your nails thinner and weaker. Furthermore, rapid abrasion of the nail surface can actually generate heat, which in turn leads to nail brittleness.

Healthy, moisturized nails have a natural, subtle shine without being buffed. If you wish to add more shine, rub your nails with a nourishing oil such as butter, vitamin E oil, fish oil or olive oil; or you can even try coating them with petroleum jelly.

That said, if you do decide to buff your nails, do it no more than once a month, and use the buffer gently. Plastic nail-buffing tools can be bought from cosmetics stores, drugstores and pharmacies.

Nail-buffing creams are another product available on the market. If you decide to use them, carefully check the list of ingredients on the label and avoid any that contain chemicals such as parabens.

People may buff their nails as a way of camouflaging an uneven nail surface. To learn more on this topic, see the section 'Nail Issues: Ridges in Nails', page 173.

BEWARE OF WEARING ARTIFICIAL NAILS

Some people are unable to grow their natural nails to the length and strength they would like. Artificial nails (also known as fake nails, false nails, fashion nails, nail enhancements, or nail extensions), are augmentations for natural nails, not replacements. They can help to hide damaged, short, discolored or deformed nails, as well as protect against nail breakage and splitting. Artificial nails may also help to stop people from biting their nails

Artificial nails can be either 'tips', which are lightweight, nail-shaped plates glued on to the ends of the natural nails, or full nails, which are custom-molded in 'forms' to fit each individual nail-shape.

These fake nails are available in a variety of designs and colors. They are made from a range of materials, including (but not limited to):
- Polymethyl methacrylate acrylics
- UV Top Coat
- Fiberglass or silk wraps

Acrylic nails are made from compounds that can be flammable. When wearing them it is important to keep a safe distance from heat sources such as hairdryers or flames from barbecues and gas cooktops.

The glues used to stick artificial nails over the top of your own nails contain adhesive chemicals so strong that it is generally necessary for the manicurist to wear a face mask when using them, to avoid breathing their fumes. Some clients may experience an adverse reaction to the smell of these chemicals.

The same applies to the solvents used to remove artificial nails. These chemicals can irritate the skin around the nails and may cause dermatitis.

People who work in manicure salons are regularly exposed to chemicals such as ethyl methacrylate, toluene, dibutyl phthalate and formaldehyde. Such substances can cause contact dermatitis, asthma and other allergic reactions.

Infection can be a problem if you wear artificial nails. It can enter your body -

- if the manicurist's tools accidentally penetrate the skin
- if the manicure tools are not properly sterilized
- if your fake nails are later dislodged and pull away from your nails, leaving a pocket which is open to fungal spores and other pathogens.

Should fungus take hold underneath the fake nails, it can deform and discolor your natural nails, making them rough and thick. If the fungal infection is not treated it may progress further and in serious cases such infections can make the real nails drop off.

Tips to decrease the health risks of artificial nails

Applying, wearing and removing artificial nails all carry health risks and we recommend that you avoid these processes However, if you do want to use artificial nails here are some helpful hints.

Minimize the covered area

Choose nail tips instead of full extensions. As a rule, nail extensions are more likely to provide a breeding ground for fungal or bacterial infections, which in extreme cases can lead to permanent damage.

Tips cover a smaller area than full extensions, so the potential home for germs is smaller.

Check for allergy-causing chemicals

Check the list of ingredients! A compound called methacrylate (MMA), which is found in some acrylic nails, has triggered such serious allergic reactions in some people that their nails have actually detached from the nail bed. This chemical is banned in several states of the USA.

It is worth asking your manicurist to use only MMA-free extensions on you.

Avoid unsterilized equipment

Manicurists in salons use their equipment on many customers If these tools are not properly sterilized, germs from one customer can be passed on to others. Make sure your manicurist follows the correct sterilization procedures. Pathogens that cause infections such as HIV, hepatitis B and hepatitis C can be transferred on dirty equipment.

Limit the number of applications

It is recommended that you do not apply artificial nails more frequently than once every three months, and that after removing the nails you allow one month to pass before new nails are attached, to give your own nails a chance to rest and heal.

Take the precaution of visiting a professional manicurist to have your artificial nails removed.

NAIL ART

The term 'nail art' refers to the decoration of nails, particularly fingernails. It includes such techniques as:

- Nail tipping
- Sculptured nails
- Nail wrapping
- Acrylic overlays
- Stickers
- Nail piercing
- Water marbling
- 3D stick-ons

Nail polish can be applied and embellished in numerous styles, such as the 'French manicure', in which the fingernails are painted pale pink with a white band across the tip, or with special effects such as sparkles, airbrushing, or glued-on gems, rhinestones and '3D' art.

BASIC FINGERNAIL AND TOENAIL CARE KIT

Equipment that can help you keep your nails healthy includes:

- Sharp nail clippers or manicure scissors
- Moisturizer
- A fine-grained nail file
- Nail brush
- Cotton-lined gloves

NAIL ISSUES: RIDGES IN NAILS

As we age, our bodies may not digest nutrients as efficiently as they did when we were young. When we are not absorbing the nutrients required for healthy nails, parts of the nail plate become thinner. These thinner areas look 'sunken', like tiny valleys between the ridges of stronger, thicker nail material.

People whose nail surfaces are ridged or pitted may be tempted to smooth them out using emery boards. This is not advisable. For a start, emery boards are too harsh; secondly, any form of abrasion is going to harm your nails.

Ridges in nails are really the strong, thick, healthy areas of the nail. It is the valleys between the ridges that are weaker, thinner and less healthy, whether due to problems with the nail matrix, a dietary deficiency, impaired nutrient absorption or an underlying illness.

Because the valleys are thinner and weaker, they are less resistant to damage. If you sand down the ridges to the level of the valleys, you are really removing the strong portions and reducing the nail plate to its most fragile and vulnerable state.

This is why it is not advisable to file or buff ridged nails as a way to 'improve' their appearance.

How else can ridged nails be beautified? Applying nail polish does nothing to disguise nail ridges. However you may wish to use, instead, a paste called a 'ridge-filling base coat'. This will occupy the valleys, rising up to the level of the ridges and thus creating a smooth surface without abrasion. It will also serve as 'armor' protecting the weak grooves.

Ridge-filling pastes are unlike nail polishes. Instead of coating the nail plate with a layer of material, they contain tiny particles that sink to rest in the nail valleys.

Choose cruelty-free products and always check the list of ingredients on the label. Some commercially-available base coats still contain harmful chemicals such as formaldehyde.

NAIL ISSUES: BRITTLE NAILS

Nails that are brittle will split, peel and break easily. This brittleness can be caused either by excessive dryness or excessive softness of the nail plate.

To combat excessive dryness, apply a moisturizer to your nails and cuticles every day.

To combat softness, avoid contact with harsh chemicals and acidic foods, such as lemons and oranges. Also avoid immersing your nails in hot water for prolonged periods. Wear protective gloves if necessary.

Some studies have found that if you take regular daily doses of the vitamin biotin, your nails may grow thicker and harder and have less chance of splitting.

For healthy people, a balanced diet of fresh foods is sufficient to ensure nail health. If your nails are weak, however, you could try either a biotin supplement or increasing your intake of foods rich in vitamin B, such as carrots and bananas.

Some remedies for brittle nails that do *not* work include
- eating gelatin
- eating calcium
- soaking your nails in gelatin

NAIL ISSUES: FUNGAL INFECTIONS

Fungal infections are more likely to attack your toenails than your fingernails, for two reasons. Firstly, the environment of a warm, sweaty shoe is more conducive to fungal growth, and secondly, because the fungi that infect nails[67] are the same as those that cause athlete's foot (*tinea pedis*). That said, fingernails can get fungal infections too.

To deter fungal infections from attacking your nails, keep them clean and dry. Never injure your nails by chewing them, or tearing off hangnails, because as soon as the skin is broken, fungus can enter.

Drugstores and pharmacies sell topical antifungal products that can be used to treat fungal infections of the feet. Choose one that contains clotrimazole or miconazole. If the infection invades beneath the nail, however, you will probably need to see your doctor. Only a strong, prescription-strength medication can deal with that.

Tea tree oil and orange oil have fungicidal properties and can be used to treat foot fungus.

Baking soda, (sodium bicarbonate) is sometimes used as a scrub or a foot-soak. Baking soda is not fungicidal, which is to say that it cannot actually destroy fungus. It is, nonetheless, *fungistatic*, which means it hinders fungus from proliferating. Baking soda foot soaks can also soften hard skin and calluses.

Some people use coconut oil to combat nail fungus. It contains antifungal fatty acids.

---

67   *Trichophyton rubrum syn. T. mentagrophytes, or Epidermophyton floccosum*

NAIL ISSUES: HANGNAILS

Hangnails are not really nails; neither are they ingrown nails. They are the dry, often brittle skin-flaps that appear hanging around the perimeter of your fingernails. If they get caught on something, they can be torn off and leave you with a break in your skin, exposed to potential infection.

Hangnails can have any of a number of causes, including skin irritation due to exposure to chemicals or allergens; damage from nail-biting; prolonged or frequent immersion in water, cutting or picking of the cuticles, or minor injuries. During cold weather, your skin is likely to be drier and more prone to developing hangnails.

Usually, you can fix them by simply clipping them off. Hangnails that are not looked after correctly can be a problem however, and they may lead to more serious consequences, such as bacterial, fungal or yeast infections in the skin surrounding the nail. Symptoms of infection usually include redness, swelling and soreness.

PREVENTING HANGNAILS

As a safeguard against the formation of hangnails. moisturize your hands regularly. If you bite your nails, make an effort to stop. Maintain neat and tidy nails as explained in the section 'Keep Nails Trimmed', page 166.

TREATING HANGNAILS

If you have a hangnail, soften it by soaking your finger (or toe) in warm water for a few minutes. Next, snip it off cleanly with a sharp pair of nail scissor or cutters. Apply a gently antiseptic or antibacterial cream and massage it into the nail bed.

If the wound from removing the hangnail is large or deep, cover it with a bandage until it has healed.

TREATING HANGNAIL INFECTIONS

Any redness, swelling, pus or soreness around the site of a hangnail probably indicates an infection. If antiseptic lotions and creams do not provide improvement, see your doctor.

NAIL ISSUES: INGROWN NAILS

If the corner of one of your nails curls around and starts to grow down into the soft tissue of your nail bed, it becomes what is known as an 'ingrown nail'. These develop more frequently on toes than on fingers.

Ingrown nails may not strictly be a beauty issue, but they are painful and usually cause inflammation. To treat this problem, trim the nail straight across the top and gently roll back the overgrown skin at the border of the ingrown nail. See if you can insert a length of dental floss beneath the nail to carefully raise it a little way away from the skin.

Try soaking the affected toe or finger every day for 15 to 20 minutes in any one of the following solutions:
- ¼ cup white vinegar in 1 cup warm water;
- 2 tablespoons Epsom salts in 4 cups warm water
- ¼ teaspoon salt in 1 cup warm water

If symptoms persist, seek treatment from your doctor or podiatrist.

NUTRITION FOR HAIR, SKIN, TEETH AND NAILS

COLLAGEN SUPPORT: SILICON AND VITAMIN C

Collagen is the main structural protein in our bodies and is important for the health of hair, skin and nails. The nutrients that help the body produce collagen include silicon and vitamin C.

Silicon may also help the body to harden tooth enamel, strengthen the gums, hair and nails, and stimulate the formation of new cells. This important nutrient is found in many foods, including vegetables, sunflower seeds, strawberries, avocados, many vegetables, and cereals. It is also available in supplement form from pharmacies/drugstores.

NUTRITION FOR NAILS AND HAIR: BIOTIN

Biotin deficiency is a rare condition; however, people who suffer from it may experience brittle nails and hair loss. If you have been diagnosed with a lack of biotin, taking the recommended dosage of 2.5 mg, per day can repair your nails and reverse hair loss. Too much biotin can seriously harm your health, so correct dosages should be strictly adhered to.

NUTRITION FOR NAILS AND HAIR: ZINC

A zinc deficiency can also slow the growth of the skin, nails and hair. In fact, it can lead to hangnails, cuticle inflammation, white spots on fingernails, poor nail growth, hair loss, skin rashes, eczema and more. Again, if you are taking zinc supplements it is vital to adhere to the correct dosage to avoid harmful overdose.

NUTRITION FOR NAILS AND HAIR: IRON

An iron deficiency can impair the growth of your hair. It can also cause 'koilonychia,' or misshapen fingernails.

EAT WELL FOR BEAUTY

Eating a wide range of fresh foods including fruits and vegetables should provide you with all the right nutrients for healthy hair, skin, teeth and nails.

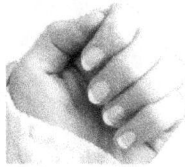

Part 8:
Home-Made
Hair Care & Toothpaste
Recipes

HOME-MADE HAIR CARE RECIPES

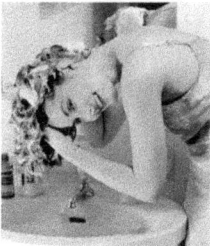

Here are some recipes for soap-free home-made shampoo and conditioners. They're simple to make, they really work and they won't break the bank. In fact, they're probably cheaper than most commercial shampoos and conditioners!

The shampoos are pH balanced. Your skin's sebum and your scalp's pH are naturally slightly acidic—between 4.5 and 5.5. This balance is vital for a healthy scalp.

Too alkaline, and the scalp becomes a breeding ground for fungi or bacteria.

Do not expect your home-made shampoos to lather up as a commercial shampoo would do. They are still cleaning your heir, even without bubbles and suds.

Never use baking soda to wash your hair—it is far too alkaline and can damage and dry out the hair if used over a prolonged period. Castile soap too, sometimes recommended for hair-washing, is highly alkaline.

If you're already using a 'natural' shampoo, check the ingredients on the label. Commercial products often contain chemical additives that are far from natural and some, such as sodium lauryl sulfate, can actually be damaging.

A NOTE ON PERFUMES AND FRAGRANCES

Perfumes and fragrances can irritate one's airways. Add to this the potential of many essential oils to irritate sensitive skin, and you have two good reasons to avoid adding perfumes and essential oils to your home-made personal care products.

HOME-MADE HAIR CARE RECIPES:

GLYCERIN AND ALOE VERA SHAMPOO

Aloe vera and vegetable glycerin both have a neutral pH of 7. Use pure aloe vera gel with no additives.

Ingredients:
- ¼ cup of pure aloe vera gel
- ¼ cup vegetable glycerin
- ½ cup water

Instructions:
- Mix together the glycerin and the aloe vera gel until the shampoo is smooth and lump-free.

To use:
- Wet your hair and massage the shampoo into your scalp.
- Allow it to remain on your hair for a couple of minutes.
- Use lukewarm water to rinse it off completely.

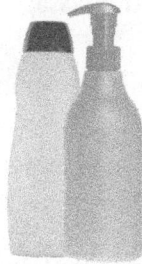

HOME-MADE HAIR CARE RECIPES:

COCONUT MILK AND ALOE VERA SHAMPOO

This recipe is excellent for dry, dandruff-prone hair and scalps. There are no preservatives in the formula so make small batches and use them within a week, or else freeze the shampoo.

To freeze, make double or triple the quantity of shampoo shown here, then pour it into ice-cube trays and store it in the freezer for later use. The night before you want to use it, simply leave aa cube or two in a covered cup at room temperature, to defrost.

Ingredients:

- 2.5 oz. (75 ml) coconut milk
- 3 oz. (90 ml) pure aloe vera gel
- Optional extras for very dry hair: a few drops of jojoba oil, vitamin E oil or sweet almond oil

Instructions:

- Mix together the coconut milk and the aloe vera gel until the shampoo is smooth and lump-free.

To use:

- Wet your hair and massage the shampoo into your scalp.
- Allow it to remain on your hair for a couple of minutes.
- Rinse it off completely, with lukewarm water.

HOME-MADE HAIR CARE RECIPES:

HAIR CONDITIONER

Ingredients:

- 1 teaspoon (5 ml) jojoba oil or virgin coconut oil (if your hair is oily, use grapeseed oil instead.)
- 1 teaspoon (5 ml) vegetable glycerin
- 1 tablespoon (8 g) emulsifying wax[68]
- ½ tsp (1.5 ml) vitamin E oil[69]
- ½ cup (125 ml) water
- 5 drops grapefruit seed extract

---

68   Emulsifying wax is a compound that is used to prevent ingredients from separating. It is available from soap-making suppliers.
69   Or two vitamin E capsules, squeezed out.

Equipment:
- A double boiler [70]
- A wooden spoon for stirring
- A separate saucepan (or a bowl if you have a microwave)
- A wire whisk
- A clean, sterilized[71] 8 oz (250 ml) dark glass bottle with lid

Instructions:
Put the oil, emulsifying wax and glycerin in the top pan of a double boiler, and add several cups of water to the lower pan. Make sure the water level does not reach high enough to touch the bottom of the top pan. Place the double boiler on your stovetop.

Turn the stovetop on to a low heat and warm the water slowly, stirring the ingredients until the wax is melted and all ingredients are well-blended.

Remove the double boiler from the stovetop and add the vitamin E oil.

Warm up the water in a separate saucepan, or in a bowl in the microwave. Make sure it is only lukewarm—not too hot. This is an important step that helps with proper emulsification.

---

70   *If you do not have a double boiler, take a bowl made of glass, Pyrex or metal) and sit it on top of a saucepan. The two should fit tightly together without any gaps between the bowl and the saucepan, and the bowl should sit partly down inside the saucepan, for good stability.*

71   *To sterilize empty bottles and their lids, stand them on a wire rack in large saucepan. Fill the saucepan and bottles with hot (not boiling) water to 1 inch (2 ½ cm) above the tops of the bottles. Bring to the boil and boil for 10 minutes. Carefully remove the hot bottles and lids one at a time and drain them.*

Gradually pour the warmed water into the oil mixture, beating constantly with a wire whisk. Continue whisking until the mixture is smooth and creamy. Let the mixture cool for a few minutes. As it cool, it will start to thicken.

Add the grapefruit seed extract and stir well.

Pour the conditioner into the sterilized dark glass bottle and allow it to cool before putting the lid on.

As the mixture cools down, shake the bottle from time to time, so that the ingredients won't separate.

Store in the refrigerator.

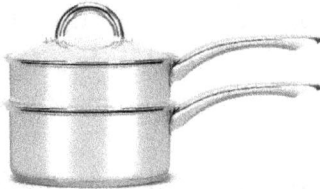

HOME-MADE HAIR CARE RECIPES:

HYPOALLERGENIC LEAVE-IN CONDITIONER

Glycerin is a humectant, which means it attracts water. When you mix it with water, it makes a great moisturizer for the hair. This mixture makes an excellent hair detangler and, if applied to the ends of the hair shaft, reduces the risk of split ends.

Simply whisk together 2 teaspoons vegetable glycerin and 1 cup water. Add an extra teaspoon of glycerin if your hair is very dry.

Make up this recipe in small batches, store in a sealed container in the fridge, and use it within a week, because it contains no preservatives.

HOME-MADE HAIR CARE RECIPES:

APPLE CIDER VINEGAR HAIR RINSE

When we shampoo our hair, the cuticles on the hair shaft cease to lie flat and overlap smoothly. Instead they open up. When this happens the hair no longer feels smooth and looks shiny. It becomes coarse and brittle, and looks dull.

Rinsing the hair with vinegar removes shampoo and other residues from the hair shafts and makes the cuticles lie flat again. This means the hair looks shinier and is less prone to become tangled or to break.

The recipe is very easy: simply mix ¼ cup to 1 cup of apple cider vinegar with 2 cups of water. If your hair is oily, use more vinegar; if dry, use less.

Store it in a plastic squeeze bottle to make it easier to apply.

After you shampoo your hair, apply generous amounts of the vinegar-water solution. Work it into your scalp and allow it to remain for a minute or two before rinsing it off with warm water.

We recommend that you use this rinse no more than twice a week, as over-use may dry out the hair.

SWEET-SCENTED VARIATIONS:

Add sweet-smelling herbs, fresh or dried, to this recipe— whole herbs, not essential oils. Choose aromatic plants such as rosemary, lavender, lemon verbena and rose geranium. Make sure they have not been sprayed with insecticides.

Ingredients:

- 2 tablespoons apple cider vinegar
- 1 cup chopped aromatic plants
- 2 cups boiling water

Instructions

In a small saucepan bring the water to the boil, then add the herbs and vinegar. Allow the herbs to simmer for a few minutes then turn off the heat, cover the saucepan with a lid and let the infusion stand for 30 minutes.

After it has cooled, pour it through a fine strainer (such as a coffee filter) and discard the herbs. Use the conditioner immediately or store it in the refrigerator and use it within the next few days.

HOME-MADE TOOTHPASTE RECIPES:

COCONUT OIL & BAKING SODA

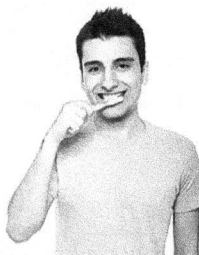

Coconut oil has antibacterial, antimicrobial, and antifungal properties, while baking soda is a very mild abrasive which helps remove debris from the teeth.

The taste of this mixture is somewhat bland. Some people sweeten it with stevia and flavor it with essential oils; however we do not recommend the use of essential oils in toothpaste.

Ingredients
- 2 tablespoons coconut oil
- 2 tablespoons baking soda

Instructions

- Whip the ingredients together in a bowl until they make a paste.
- Pour into a glass jar with a lid, for storage.

Thank you for reading this book!

If you have found value in our beauty books, please review them on Amazon and Goodreads. It would mean the world to us!

The Team at Leaves of Gold Press.

About the author:

Elizabeth Reed is a university graduate and author with an interest in researching the 'science of beauty'. She spent a year writing the 'Beauty' series, examining studies from across the globe. She lives with her husband in Australia, and is the mother of three children.

IS
FOOD
MAKING YOU
SICK?

With more than 100 recipes

The
Strictly Low Histamine Diet

ECZEMA sleep disorders REFLUX *nausea* anxiety
SINUSITIS stomach PAIN *fuzzy* thinking *itching*
joint pain irritability *hives* HEADACHES bowel DISEASE
asthma
inflammation hayfever DIZZINESS diarrhea *migraines*

and more . . .

James L. Gibb

IS FOOD MAKING YOU SICK?

THE STRICTLY LOW HISTAMINE DIET

By James L. Gibb

People all over the world suffer from histamine intolerance without being aware of it.

The symptoms are many and widely varied, often resembling food allergies or other diseases. They can affect the digestive system, the respiratory system, the skin and many other parts of the body. These problems may endure throughout our entire lives if we continue to consume large amounts of histamine.

Histamine is colorless, odorless and tasteless - undetectable except by scientific analysis, and yet crucial to our well-being.

Individual histamine tolerance thresholds vary greatly. A range of circumstances including our genes, our environment, our diet and stress, cause our bodies' histamine levels to rise.
If they rise faster than our bodies can break them down, we experience the excessive inflammation brought on by histamine intolerance, or HIT.

The good news is, if we can understand what is happening and why, we can treat or prevent this widely unrecognized but very real condition.

Index

C

F

G

H

R

S

ABOUT THE AUTHOR

Elizabeth Reed is a university graduate and author with an interest in researching the 'science of beauty'. She spent a year writing the 'Beauty' series, examining studies from across the globe and physically undergoing some of the less invasive— though not necessarily less painful—cosmetic treatments, largely so that she could report on them from first hand experience. She lives with her husband in Australia, and is the mother of three children.

Also from Leaves of Gold Press:

THE NEW BESTSELLER

IS

FOOD

MAKING YOU

SICK?

With more than 100 recipes

The
Strictly Low Histamine Diet

ECZEMA sleep disorders   REFLUX *nausea* anxiety
SINUSITIS stomach PAIN *fuzzy* thinking *itching*
joint pain irritability *hives* HEADACHES bowel DISEASE
asthma
inflammation hayfever DIZZINESS diarrhea *migraines*

and more . . .

James L. Gibb

IS FOOD MAKING YOU SICK?

THE STRICTLY LOW HISTAMINE DIET

By James L. Gibb

People all over the world suffer from histamine intolerance without being aware of it.

The symptoms are many and widely varied, often resembling food allergies or other diseases. They can affect the digestive system, the respiratory system, the skin and many other parts of the body. These problems may endure throughout our entire lives if we continue to consume large amounts of histamine.

Histamine is colorless, odorless and tasteless - undetectable except by scientific analysis, and yet crucial to our well-being.

Individual histamine tolerance thresholds vary greatly. A range of circumstances including our genes, our environment, our diet and stress, cause our bodies' histamine levels to rise.

If they rise faster than our bodies can break them down, we experience the excessive inflammation brought on by histamine intolerance, or HIT.

The good news is, if we can understand what is happening and why, we can treat or prevent this widely unrecognized but very real condition.

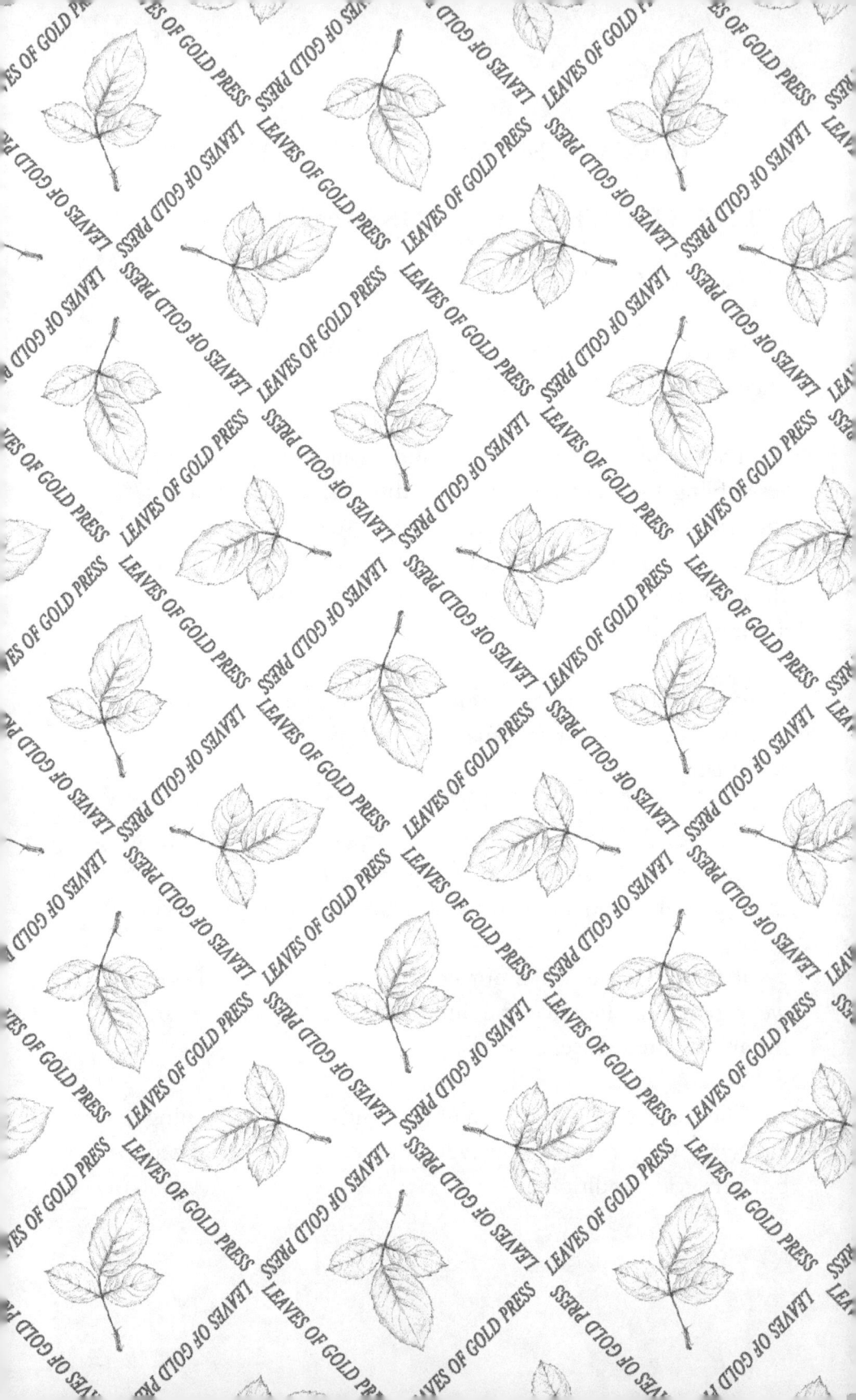

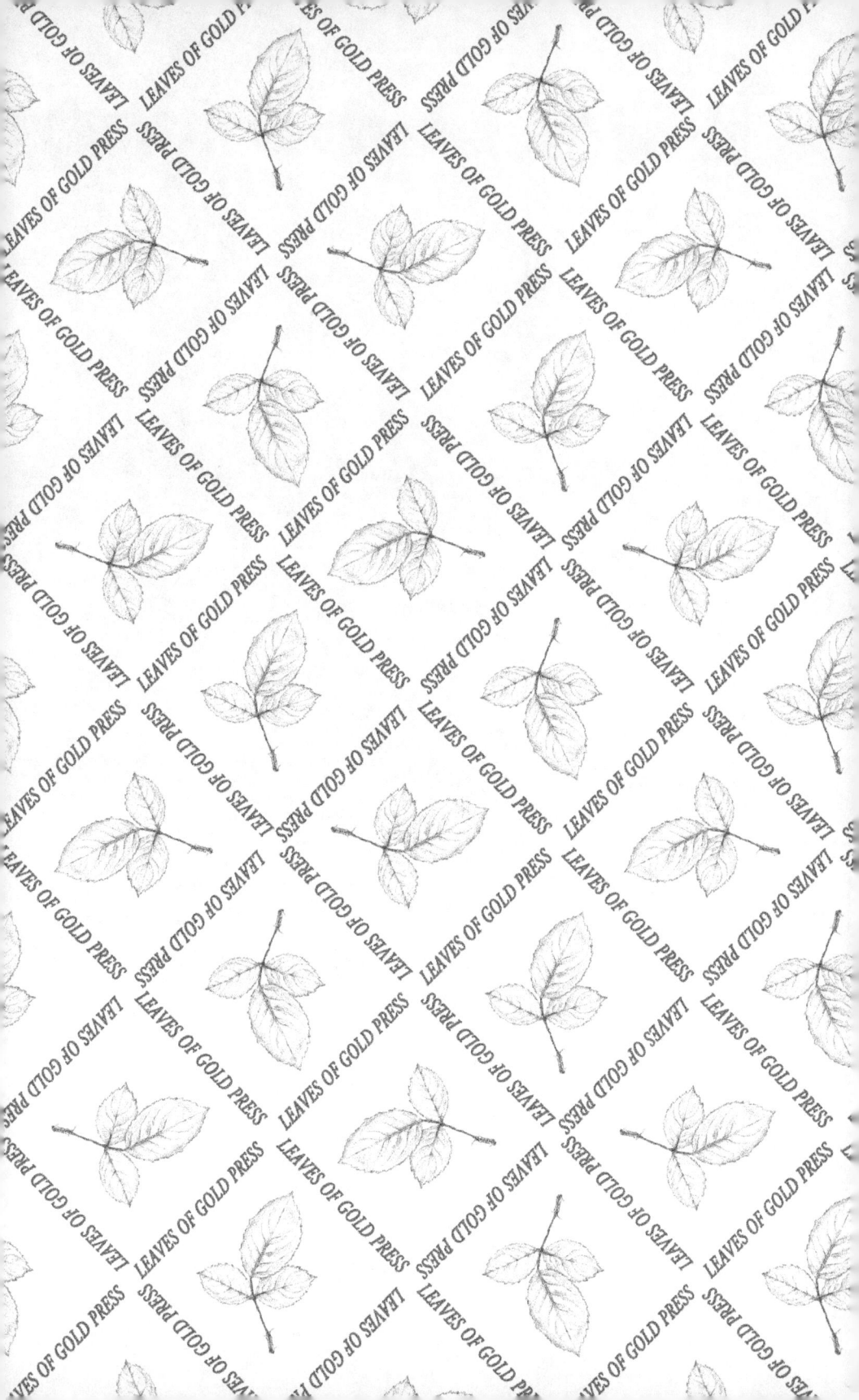